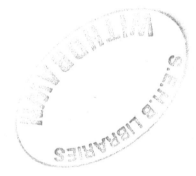

Negative Symptom and Cognitive Deficit Treatment Response in Schizophrenia

Negative Symptom and Cognitive Deficit Treatment Response in Schizophrenia

Edited by

RICHARD S. E. KEEFE, PH.D.
JOSEPH P. MCEVOY, M.D.

American
Psychiatric
Press, Inc.

Washington, DC
London, England

Note: The authors have worked to ensure that all information in this book concerning drug dosages, schedules, and routes of administration is accurate as of the time of publication and consistent with standards set by the U.S. Food and Drug Administration and the general medical community. As medical research and practice advance, however, therapeutic standards may change. For this reason and because human and mechanical errors sometimes occur, we recommend that readers follow the advice of a physician who is directly involved in their care or the care of a member of their family.

Copyright © 2001 American Psychiatric Press, Inc.
ALL RIGHTS RESERVED
Manufactured in the United States of America on acid-free paper
04 03 02 01   4 3 2 1
First Edition

American Psychiatric Press, Inc.
1400 K Street, N.W., Washington, DC 20005
www.appi.org

Library of Congress Cataloging-in-Publication Data
Negative symptom and cognitive deficit treatment response in schizophrenia / edited by Richard S. E. Keefe, Joseph P. McEvoy. – 1st ed.
        p. ; cm.
Includes bibliographic references and index.
ISBN 0-88048-785-2 (alk. paper)
        1. Schizophrenia–Diagnosis. 2. Schizophrenia–Chemotherapy.
3. Cognition disorders–Chemotherapy. I. Keefe, Richard S. E.
II. McEvoy, Joseph P., 1948-
        [DNLM: 1. Schizophrenia–drug therapy. 2. Antipsychotic Agents–
therapeutic use. 3. Cognition Disorders–drug therapy. 4. Schizophrenia–
diagnosis. 5. Schizophrenia Psychology. 6. Treatment Outcome.
WM 203 A846 2000]
RC514 .A79 2000
616.89'82–dc21

                                                                00-023099

British Library Cataloguing in Publication Data
A CIP record is available from the British Library.

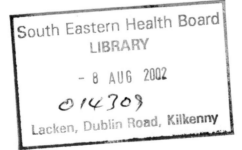

Contents

Contributors

Xavier F. Amador, Ph.D.
Director, Department of Psychology, New York State Psychiatric Institute, and Associate Professor in Psychology, College of Physicians and Surgeons and Teacher's College, Columbia University, New York, New York

Nancy C. Andreasen, M.D., Ph.D.
Director, Mental Health Clinical Research Center and PET Imaging Center, The University of Iowa College of Medicine and Hospitals and Clinics, Iowa City, Iowa

Paul Bailey, M.R.C.Psych.
Research Psychiatrist, FORENAP (Foundation for Research in Neuroscience Applied to Psychiatry), Centre Hospitalier, Rouffach, France

Robert W. Buchanan, M.D.
Chief, Outpatient Research Program, Maryland Psychiatric Research Center, Department of Psychiatry, University of Maryland at Baltimore

William T. Carpenter Jr., M.D.
Director, Maryland Psychiatric Research Center, Department of Psychiatry, University of Maryland at Baltimore

Michael Flaum, M.D.
Associate Professor, Mental Health Clinical Research Center, The University of Iowa College of Medicine and Hospitals and Clinics, Iowa City, Iowa

Dale L. Johnson, Ph.D.
Professor, Department of Psychology, University of Houston, Houston, Texas

Richard S. E. Keefe, Ph.D.
Associate Professor, Department of Psychiatry and Behavioral Sciences, Duke University Medical Center, Durham, North Carolina

Christie Limpert, Ph.D.
Associate Psychologist, Bronx Children's Psychiatric Center, Bronx, New York

Jean-Pierre Lindenmayer, M.D.
Director, Psychopharmacology Research Unit, Manhattan Psychiatric Center, Nathan Kline Institute for Psychiatric Research, and Clinical Professor, Department of Psychiatry, New York University School of Medicine, New York, New York

Joseph P. McEvoy, M.D.
Associate Professor, Department of Psychiatry and Behavioral Sciences, Duke University Medical Center, Durham, North Carolina

Del D. Miller, Pharm.D., M.D.
Associate Professor of Psychiatry, Department of Psychiatry, and Director, Neuropsychiatry Unit, Mental Health Clinical Research Center, The University of Iowa Hospitals and Clinics, Iowa City, Iowa

Kim T. Mueser, Ph.D.
Professor, Department of Psychiatry, Dartmouth Medical School, Lebanon, New Hampshire

Peg Nopoulos, M.D.
Clinical Director, Mental Health Clinical Research Center, The University of Iowa College of Medicine and Hospitals and Clinics, Iowa City, Iowa

Rajiv Tandon, M.D.
Professor of Psychiatry, Department of Psychiatry; Director, Hospital Services
Division; and Director, Schizophrenia Program, University of Michigan
Medical Center, Ann Arbor, Michigan

Susan L. Trumbetta, Ph.D.
Assistant Professor, Department of Psychology, Vassar College, Poughkeepsie,
New York

Introduction

Richard S. E. Keefe, Ph.D.
Joseph P. McEvoy, M.D.

Negative symptoms have become increasingly important in the diagnosis and treatment of schizophrenia. Not only were negative symptoms included for the first time as a criterion for the diagnosis of schizophrenia in DSM-IV (American Psychiatric Association 1994), but atypical antipsychotic medications for schizophrenia, such as clozapine, risperidone, and olanzapine, are purported to have specific effects on negative symptoms and cognitive dysfunction. However, many controversies relating to the assessment of these symptoms have prevented researchers from drawing clear conclusions about the efficacy of these treatments, and these areas of conflict often prevent clinicians from making clear determinations about the treatment response of individual patients. This book describes the latest research on the assessment of negative symptoms and cognitive dysfunction for the purposes of evaluating treatment efficacy in research studies and determining individual treatment response in clinical practice.

A variety of different approaches to defining—and assessing the effects of treatment on—schizophrenia symptoms have been developed in recent years. The understanding of treatment response in different symptom domains in schizophrenia has been advanced by these conceptualizations and the assessment instruments that have sprung from them. However, as is clear from the varying methodologies used and the contradictory results reported by studies of negative symptom response to typical and atypical antipsychotics (reviewed by Lindenmayer in Chapter 4), no consensus has been reached regarding the best methods for assessing negative symptom treatment response—or even for the definition of adequate response. In addition, as discussed by Bailey in Chapter 8, no drug has been licensed specifically for the indication of negative symptom treatment, and the criteria for this indication have not been established. The negative symptoms that have been assessed and the instruments that have been used to measure negative symptom treatment response have varied considerably from study to study. Furthermore, the relationship between extrapyramidal side effects and negative symptom variation as a result of pharmacological treatment has only recently begun to be explored—yet elucidation of this relationship is sorely needed. These issues are complex and are addressed fully in this volume.

One of the primary difficulties faced in evaluating negative symptom treatment response is that whereas many of the instruments currently in use for assessing treatment outcome have significant strengths, none stands out as clearly better than any other. Thus, the decision to use a particular scale in a particular trial is either arbitrary or the result of a compromise between competing needs. As a consequence, results from different research centers addressing the same question are not comparable. In his comparison of seven negative symptom rating scales, Lindenmayer (Chapter 4) notes that although the reliability of all of these scales is fair to good, the temporal stability of negative symptoms varies tremendously depending on which scale is used. He also points out that current conceptions of and assessment methods for negative symptoms vary tremendously, with often very little overlap. Instruments differ substantially regarding the symptoms assessed, the scaling of the items in terms of frequency or severity of behaviors, the time period over which symptoms are measured, and the relative emphasis on observed behaviors versus subjective complaints. Because these instruments were not designed specifically for treatment trials, little is known about their reliability, validity, and sensitivity in assessing negative symptom treatment response. Development of an assessment tool with a broad range of symptom dimensions and a high degree of sensitivity to drug-associated changes that could be used by multiple investigators evaluating the same issues would facilitate clearer communication regarding treatment responsivity in schizophrenia. Although a consensus agreement to use a particular instrument has not been achieved in this area of schizophrenia research, such agreements have been reached in other medical disciplines and for some other psychiatric disorders.

Many important sources of information regarding negative symptom improvement or worsening are often ignored. In Chapter 7, Johnson discusses the use of information from family members of those with schizophrenia and the impact of negative symptoms on relatives of schizophrenic patients. He calls for the development of specific family-oriented scales to assess negative symptoms in clinical trials and other scientific research. Limpert and Amador, the authors of Chapter 6, emphasize the importance of measuring the *experience* of emotion in patients with schizophrenia and explain how this subjective aspect of negative symptoms differs from the more traditional objectively measured facets of these symptoms. They argue that deficits in emotional experiencing may remain refractory to improvement even in otherwise treatment-responsive patients.

The measurement of negative symptom treatment response can be thwarted by confounding factors, such as extrapyramidal side effects of medications, depressive symptoms, and psychotic (positive) symptoms, all of which can mimic negative symptoms. In Chapter 2, Nopoulos and colleagues discuss strategies for disentangling primary negative symptoms from negative symptoms that are secondary to other etiologies. It is important to note that eliminating one confound (e.g., discontinuing antipsychotic medication to eliminate extrapyramidal side effects) can enhance another confound (e.g., exacerbating psychosis and thereby potentially worsening negative symptoms). Although statistical corrections and careful experimental design can reduce these confounds, they cannot eliminate them completely.

In attempting to determine the best method for assessing negative symptom treatment response, it is important to distinguish between negative symptoms and "deficit" symptoms. As described by Buchanan and Carpenter in Chapter 1, the *deficit syndrome* is characterized by a pattern of enduring negative symptoms that persist in an individual for at least 1 year and that are not secondary to factors such as depression, medication side effects, anxiety, delusions, and hallucinations. With regard to this construct, a key question addressed by these authors is whether "pure" negative–or deficit–symptoms respond to treatment with atypical antipsychotics, low-dose typical antipsychotics, or behavioral interventions. Buchanan and Carpenter also present guidelines for the treatment of patients with negative symptoms.

The effect of treatment on social functioning and subjective experience of quality of life is likely to be evident only after a time period that extends beyond the traditional treatment response study. Patients with neurocognitive deficits who have been delusional and hallucinating for extended periods of time prior to treatment may have become socially isolated and may be functioning substantially below their original level. Although these patients may never return to their baseline level of social functioning, even small improvements in socialization may be extremely important to their quality of life, and are worthy of assessment. These changes, however, may not occur during a typical 6- to 8-week drug treatment trial and will require assessment beyond this period of time. It is likely that in some patients, social functioning will improve only after a reduction in positive symptoms, medication side effects, certain negative symptoms, and cognitive dysfunction that can be ameliorated with drug treatment. As discussed by Trumbetta and Mueser in Chapter 3, the course of social deficits is complex and is greatly affected by premorbid social development, age at illness onset, and other symptom domains. These authors suggest that behavioral interventions may be excellent adjuncts to pharmacological treatment for the improvement of social deficits in schizophrenia patients.

Although cognitive impairment is not one of the the criteria for schizophrenia, most schizophrenic patients demonstrate cognitive deficits in a variety of areas, including abstraction, attention, language, and memory. These cognitive deficits are strongly correlated with poor community functioning and unemployment. In Chapter 3, Trumbetta and Mueser describe the importance of neurocognitive dysfunction in the social deficits of schizophrenia. With typical antipsychotic treatment, many of these impairments persist despite significant amelioration of other symptoms. As discussed by Keefe in Chapter 5, novel antipsychotics appear to improve cognitive function and may ameliorate negative symptoms through neurocognitive mechanisms. Thus, enhancement of cognitive functioning may play a major role in improving the quality of patients' lives. Specific guidelines for assessing neurocognitive treatment response are outlined by Keefe in his chapter.

Finally, what is currently known about the biological underpinnings of negative symptom treatment response? In Chapter 9, Miller and Tandon review the most recent research on the neurobiology of negative symptoms, focusing on the role of various neurotransmitter systems and various brain regions in mediating negative symptom pathology. They suggest that whereas the possibility remains that a single pathophysiological pathway mediates negative symptoms, different etiological factors may all produce negative symptoms via multiple pathophysiological processes. They raise the question of whether a single treatment modality is effective for alleviating negative symptoms, or whether distinct treatments may be effective in treating different aspects of negative symptoms.

Despite the obvious importance of these issues to the assessment of negative symptom treatment response, they are rarely addressed directly in empirical studies of patients with schizophrenia and have never before been the subject of an entire edited volume such as this. This book is intended for all clinicians who treat patients with schizophrenia and who want to know and document whether their interventions ameliorate negative symptoms and cognitive dysfunction, as well as for all researchers studying schizophrenia, particularly those interested in clinical issues and treatment studies.

1

Evaluating Negative Symptom Treatment Efficacy

Robert W. Buchanan, M.D.
William T. Carpenter Jr., M.D.

The construct of primary negative symptoms is central to the understanding of schizophrenia. This aspect of schizophrenia psychopathology has proven to be independent from hallucinations, delusions, and disorganized behavior (Buchanan and Carpenter 1994); is a robust predictor of quality of life and social and occupational functioning (Buchanan and Gold 1996); is associated with a differential pattern of cognitive and neuropsychological functional abnormalities (Buchanan et al. 1994, 1997; Bustillo et al. 1997; Strauss 1993); emanates from a neural substrate different from the neural circuits subserving other aspects of this disorder (Carpenter et al. 1993; Liddle et al. 1992); and is distinguished in studies of pharmacological probes and treatments (Carpenter 1996). Primary negative symptoms also appear to have a unique pattern of associations with etiological risk factors (e.g., genetics, season of birth, Borna disease virus; see Dworkin et al. 1988; Kendler et al. 1986; Kirkpatrick et al. 1998; Waltrip et al. 1997).

Development of an effective treatment for primary negative symptoms is now a leading therapeutic challenge for clinicians. However, our ability to critically evaluate proposed treatments is compromised by important conceptual methodological limitations. In this chapter, we review the major methodological issues involved in treating patients with negative symptoms and conducting negative symptom clinical trials, use the clozapine experience as

Supported in part by Grants MH40279 and MH45074 from the National Institute of Mental Health.

an illustration of these issues, critique current attempts to deal with these issues, and conclude with recommendations for the treatment of the patient with negative symptoms and for the optimal design of clinical trials.

We begin with two general statements concerning theory and treatment. These statements will make explicit our underlying conceptual positions and provide the foundation for the subsequent discussion.

Statement on Theory

Negative symptoms are important clinical features of schizophrenia, but it is only the primary form of these symptoms that is relevant to disease etiology and pathophysiology. This form of negative symptoms is derived from Kraepelin's (1919/1971) description of avolitional pathology and is operationalized through the use of the *deficit syndrome* concept (Carpenter et al. 1988). Enduring primary negative symptoms are referred to as *deficit symptoms* and meet specific criteria for primary disease trait manifestations (Kirkpatrick et al. 1989). The distinction between deficit and secondary negative symptoms is made reliably (Kirkpatrick et al. 1989) and is essential to any investigation in which negative symptom hypotheses are derived from schizophrenia theory.

Statement on Treatment

Patients with schizophrenia are frequently characterized by the presence of negative symptoms, as assessed with commonly used rating scales. During periods of symptom exacerbation or relapse, patients will often exhibit a concurrent increase in positive and negative symptom ratings. As patients recover from psychotic episodes, either spontaneously or with treatment, a reduction is typically seen in negative symptom ratings. In patients treated with either conventional or novel antipsychotics, it has been argued that this reduction in negative symptom ratings demonstrates the drug's negative symptom efficacy and potentially represents its effect on *primary* negative symptoms (Beasley et al. 1996; Goldberg 1985; Kane et al. 1988; Marder and Meibach 1994). We would suggest that the data require a more cautious interpretation, for two reasons. First, some of the rating scale items used to assess negative symptoms are actually measures of general psychopathology. As a result, changes in ratings for these items could reflect nonspecific improvement in global function as psychosis is reduced rather than improvement specific to the avolitional component of the illness. Second, because negative symptom ratings routinely include both primary negative and secondary negative symptoms, observed changes in negative symptom ratings could simply reflect improvement in secondary negative symptoms. To the extent that these considerations either partly or completely explain observed negative symptom improvement, any inference regarding change in primary negative symptoms is undermined.

Methodological Issues

Issue 1. Which symptoms should be included in the assessment of negative symptoms?

Although there is generally widespread agreement that negative symptoms represent diminished normal functioning (Berrios 1985), there is considerably less agreement about which symptoms should be included under the rubric of negative symptoms (Fenton and McGlashan 1992; Sommers 1985). The inclusion of symptoms that have little construct validity undermines the ability of clinicians and investigators to assess the presence and evaluate the responsiveness of primary negative symptoms. For example, Goldberg (1985) argued that placebo-controlled studies support the efficacy of conventional antipsychotics for negative and deficit symptoms. However, he included hebephrenic (i.e., disorganization) symptoms as negative symptoms. These symptoms have limited face validity as negative symptoms, and a large empirical database further serves to document their low construct validity (Andreasen et al. 1995; Buchanan and Carpenter 1994).

This issue is also encountered in scales specifically designed to assess negative symptoms. The Scale for the Assessment of Negative Symptoms (SANS; Andreasen 1982) assesses five symptom areas: affective flattening, alogia, avolition/apathy, anhedonia/asociality, and attention. However, studies have suggested that inappropriate affect, which is included as part of affective flattening; poverty of content of speech, which is included as part of alogia; and attentional symptoms may not be sufficiently associated with negative symptomatology to warrant their continued inclusion on the scale (for a review, see Buchanan and Carpenter 1994). Similarly, the Positive and Negative Syndrome Scale (PANSS; Kay et al. 1987) includes two items, Difficulty in Abstract Thinking and Stereotyped Thinking, that are designed to assess cognitive functions hypothesized to be associated with negative symptoms. However, the alpha coefficient for the PANSS negative subscale is increased when these items are deleted (Kay et al. 1987), which, in combination with their failure to load on the negative symptom factor with PANSS items (Kay and Sevy 1990), suggests that they have limited construct validity.

It is our assertion that in assessments made for the purpose of evaluating the negative symptom efficacy of a drug, only symptoms for which there is a broad basis of agreement should be used. Two possible approaches may be used to guide the selection of appropriate symptoms. First, a review of extant negative symptom rating scales reveals that only affective flattening and poverty of speech are uniformly included in these scales (Fenton and McGlashan 1992). The broad agreement on the inclusion of these two items supports their construct validity. Second, a large number of studies have examined, through the use of factor analytic techniques, the relationships among symptoms observed in patients with schizophrenia (Andreasen et al. 1995; Buchanan and Carpenter 1994). These studies have found that the following four symptoms consistently load on the negative symptom factor: affective flattening, poverty of speech (alogia), avolition, and anhedonia (Buchanan and Carpenter 1994). The converging evidence from these two approaches provides an empirical foundation supporting their construct validity and argues for their use in the assessment of negative symptom drug efficacy.

Issue 2. Which rating scale items should be used to assess negative symptoms?

The second methodological issue follows from the first and concerns which items should be used in the assessment of these symptoms. To the extent that individual scale items are unrelated or only distantly related to the negative symptom construct they are intended to measure, they will introduce unwanted variance into the assessment of these symptoms. This problem can be demonstrated in almost any rating scale currently used for the assessment of negative symptoms. Factor 2 (emotional withdrawal, motor retardation, and blunted affect) of the Brief Psychiatric Rating Scale (BPRS; Lukoff et al. 1986) has been extensively used as a proxy measure for negative symptoms. Although blunted affect is routinely accepted as a negative symptom, emotional withdrawal, which refers to a deficiency in relating to the interviewer and to the interview situation, and motor retardation, which refers to a reduction in energy level evidenced in slowed movements, are more problematic. The negative symptom construct underlying diminished social behavior (i.e., asocial behavior) is loss of social drive (Carpenter et al. 1988; Kirkpatrick and Buchanan 1990; Kirkpatrick et al. 1989). Loss of social drive is only one of several mechanisms that may underlie decreased relatedness to the interviewer. Patients may be emotionally withdrawn because they are paranoid or because they are overwhelmed by their hallucinations and delusions and withdraw as a defensive maneuver to minimize external stimuli and/or decrease the stress on their disorganized cognitive processes (Carpenter et al. 1985). Motor retardation is a vegetative sign observed in patients with depression as well as in individuals who are catatonic or suffering from antipsychotic extrapyramidal side effects (EPS). It is conceptually unrelated to the negative symptom *loss of motivation* (Carpenter et al. 1988). In the SANS, the Impersistence at Work or School and the Grooming and Hygiene items are designed to assess avolition/apathy; however, these symptoms are not specific to schizophrenia; patients with cognitive impairments or disorganized behavior are also commonly observed to have difficulties in these areas (Breier et al. 1991; Green 1996).

Issue 3. Are negative symptoms primary or secondary?

The most important methodological issue in the clinical evaluation of pharmacological agents for the treatment of negative symptoms is the differentiation of primary and secondary negative symptoms. Negative symptoms may be primary and represent an intrinsic feature of schizophrenia, or they may be secondary to factors extrinsic to schizophrenia or to other intrinsic psychopathological features of schizophrenia. Extrinsic factors include medication side effects (e.g., sedation, akinesia) (Carpenter et al. 1985) and environmental deprivation (Wing and Brown 1970); other intrinsic factors include positive symptoms and dysphoric affect (Carpenter et al. 1985). Both primary negative and secondary negative symptoms may be either transient or enduring.

Case Examples

The following two case vignettes illustrate the differences between patients with primary and secondary negative symptoms.

> Mr. A is a 43-year-old man with a diagnosis of schizophrenia, undifferentiated type. He has been ill for more than 20 years and has received a broad range of pharmacological treatments. He is extremely suspicious and occasionally presents with paranoid delusions. In addition, his speech is characterized by looseness of associations. Although Mr. A denies other positive symptoms, he is frequently observed talking to himself. He is not depressed or anxious, nor does he exhibit overt EPS. He is poorly groomed, is unemployed, has a reduced social network, and has no contact with family members. His affect is blunted, and his speech is diminished in amount, with predominantly single-word replies to questions. Mr. A rarely initiates conversation. He has few interests, although he does follow several of the local

sports teams and enjoys music. Conversing with Mr. A reveals that his diminished social and occupational behavior is largely secondary to his paranoia.

Mr. A is started on a new-generation antipsychotic (he had previously been treated with the decanoate form of a conventional antipsychotic). In response to this change in treatment, his suspiciousness diminishes, his thought disorder improves, and he is no longer observed to talk to himself. Mr. A begins to take an increased interest in his personal appearance, which includes leaving his apartment to go clothes shopping. In addition, he takes on responsibility for the care of an elderly woman who lives in his apartment complex. He spends time with her, does her food shopping, and cleans her apartment. Mr. A is also less suspicious of his landlord. His affect is brighter, he makes jokes, and his speech is increased in amount and spontaneity. He states that he feels less drugged and has more energy on the new medication.

Mr. A initially presented with multiple negative symptoms, which significantly improved in association with a medication-related decrease in suspiciousness, conceptual disorganization, and sedation. The concurrent decrease in positive and negative symptoms and in medication-induced sedation support the original conceptualization of the secondary nature of his negative symptoms.

Mr. B is a 39-year-old man with a diagnosis of schizophrenia, undifferentiated type. Like Mr. A, he has been ill for 20 years. He experiences occasional auditory hallucinations but shows no evidence of delusions or disorganized behavior. He is not depressed or anxious, nor does he exhibit any evidence of EPS or sedation. In contrast to this lack of positive symptoms, Mr. B has marked negative symptoms, including flat affect, poverty of speech (his replies are usually monosyllabic, and he rarely initiates conversation), and loss of motivation and social drive. Although he attends a psychosocial rehabilitation center, he does not engage in any of the activities provided; nonetheless, he will perform a task when directed. Mr. B has no friends, nor does he have any desire to make any; his social network is restricted to his family. He prefers to be alone, but is not bored or lonely. Although he listens to the radio and watches television, he does not seem to enjoy these activities and is unable to recall what he has heard or seen. Mr. B's therapist comments, "I have never been able to see the person within him."

Mr. B's presentation remains unchanged regardless of whether he is drug-free or being treated with conventional or new-generation antipsychotics. There are no other symptoms or environmental factors that can reasonably explain his negative symptom presentation. His presentation is characteristic of a patient with the deficit syndrome.

Rating Scales Designed to Assess Primary Negative Symptoms

Secondary negative symptoms are responsive to a broad range of treatment interventions, with the specific intervention dependent on the secondary causal factor (see below). However, their inclusion in the assessment of negative symptom responsiveness will undermine the ability of clinicians to evaluate the efficacy of a drug for primary negative symptoms. Unfortunately, the majority of rating instruments make no attempt to differentiate primary negative symptoms from secondary negative symptoms. As previously described, this problem is compounded to the extent that rating scales include symptoms or items with limited construct validity.

Three rating scales–the PANSS, the Quality of Life Scale (QLS; Heinrichs et al. 1984), and the Schedule for the Deficit Syndrome (SDS; Kirkpatrick et al. 1989)–have been specifically designed to assess primary negative symptoms.

The PANSS is purportedly designed to differentiate primary from secondary negative symptoms, and most of its items are closely associated with the negative symptom construct they are intended to assess. In addition, the descriptions for several items (e.g., Passive/Apathetic Social Withdrawal and Lack of Spontaneity and Flow of Conversation) state that raters are to record the symptom as present only when it is associated with apathy and/or avolition. However, item descriptions do not provide guidance for assessing all possible secondary causes of negative symptoms, and secondary causes of the Blunted Affect or Emotional Withdrawal items are not excluded.

The QLS is composed of four groups of items: Intrapsychic Foundations, Interpersonal Relations, Instrumental Role, and Common Objects and Activities. However, despite its having been designed to assess deficit symptoms, the QLS does not specify how either the primary/secondary or the transient/ enduring distinction is to be made, nor does it indicate which of the items constitute deficit symptom items.

Formalization of the deficit syndrome construct and specification of criteria for its assessment led to the development of the SDS (Carpenter et al. 1988; Kirkpatrick et al. 1989), a semistructured interview of documented reliability designed to categorize patients as having either the deficit or the nondeficit form of schizophrenia. The instrument provides specific criteria for assessing the presence, severity, and duration of six negative symptoms and for determining whether the symptoms are primary or secondary. By definition, patients with the deficit syndrome have two or more primary and enduring negative symptoms. The "primary and enduring" criterion does not preclude these symptoms' responsiveness to pharmacological intervention; rather, the distinction is designed to parallel the similar distinction made to select patients with enduring, trait-positive symptoms for studies of clozapine in treatment-resistant patients (Breier et al. 1994; Kane et al. 1988; Pickar et al. 1992). The major limitation of the SDS, with respect to its use in clinical trials, is that it is not designed to assess change in negative symptoms. The use of the SDS–and, specifically, the application of the deficit syndrome concept–in clinical trials is described in the following section.

Issue 4. How should change in secondary causes of negative symptoms be assessed in clinical trials?

The fourth methodological issue concerns the assessment of change in secondary causes of negative symptoms during the conduct of a clinical trial. Three sources of secondary negative symptoms can be readily measured: positive symptoms, anxiety and depressive symptoms, and medication side effects, including EPS and sedation. Failure to assess the relationship between concurrent change in these variables and negative symptoms precludes accurate evaluation of a drug's efficacy for primary negative symptoms. However, the ability of clinicians to assess the extent to which observed negative symptom change is attributable to change in secondary sources of negative symptoms is limited by two factors: 1) the sensitivity and reliability of rating instruments and 2) the presence of additional causes of secondary negative symptoms (e.g., environmental deprivation) that cannot be practically assessed during the conduct of a clinical trial.

Issue 5. What is the ideal duration of a negative symptom clinical trial?

Because positive psychotic symptoms, including symptoms in treatment-resistant patients, begin their response trajectory during the first week of treatment, clinical trials lasting a few weeks are usually adequate for testing a treatment's positive symptom efficacy (Glovinsky et al. 1992; Kane et al. 1988). In contrast, because there are no known effective treatments for primary negative symptoms, the appropriate duration of a negative symptom clinical trial is less clear. If one leaves aside the question of whether negative symptom response observed in clinical trials is due to primary or secondary negative symptoms, previous experience suggests that changes in negative symptoms are delayed relative to changes in positive symptoms (Kane et al. 1988; Lieberman et al. 1994). This would suggest that a relatively longer trial would be appropriate.

A promising development in the treatment of primary negative symptoms is the use of agents (e.g., glycine, d-cycloserine, d-serine) that act at the glycine site of the N-methyl-D-aspartate (NMDA) receptor complex (Goff et al. 1995, 1999; Heresco-Levy et al. 1999; Javitt et al. 1994; Liederman et al. 1996; Tsai et al. 1998). The results of studies employing these agents suggest that significant negative symptom improvement may be evident as early as 2 weeks after the initiation of treatment (Goff et al. 1995). In double-blind trials, significant negative symptom improvement has been observed within 6–8 weeks of treatment initiation (Goff et al. 1999; Heresco-Levy et al. 1999; Javitt et al. 1994). Thus, in order to maximize the likelihood of detecting a therapeutic effect of a drug, it is our recommendation that negative symptom clinical trials be of at least 8 weeks' duration.

These five methodological issues may have a marked impact on the evaluation of the efficacy of pharmacological interventions for negative symptoms. The investigation of the efficacy of clozapine for negative symptoms highlights many of these issues.

Illustration: The Clozapine Experience

Clozapine has been found to be more effective than conventional antipsychotics for the treatment of positive symptoms in treatment-resistant patients with schizophrenia (Buchanan et al. 1998; Kane et al. 1988; Pickar et al. 1992). In a study by Kane and colleagues (1988), clozapine was also observed to have superior efficacy for negative symptoms, as assessed with BPRS Factor 2 and Disorientation items. However, in that study, it was not possible to ascertain whether this effect included improvement in primary negative symptoms, since the change in negative symptoms was associated with significant concurrent reductions in positive symptoms and EPS. In another study of inpatients with schizophrenia, both the BPRS Factor 2 and the SANS were used to assess negative symptom response (Pickar et al. 1992). A significant reduction was again observed with BPRS Factor 2, leading the authors to conclude that clozapine had superior efficacy for negative symptoms. However, as in the Kane et al. study, this change in negative symptoms occurred in the context of significant changes in positive symptoms and EPS. Moreover, a superior advantage of clozapine for negative symptoms was not detected by the SANS ratings.

A number of investigations have attempted to determine whether clozapine's observed efficacy for negative symptoms includes primary negative symptoms. In an open-labeled study, negative symptom improvement could not be entirely accounted for by changes in positive symptoms (Meltzer 1992). However, the open-label study design, the lack of a comparison group, the inclusion of symptoms with little construct validity, and the failure to take into account other sources of secondary negative symptoms precluded a primary negative symptom response interpretation (Carpenter et al. 1995). In other studies, significant correlations between changes in negative symptoms and changes in hallucinations and delusions (Lieberman et al. 1994; Tandon et al. 1993a), positive formal thought disorder (Miller et al. 1994b; Tandon et al. 1993a), and/or EPS (Lieberman et al. 1994) have been observed.

Two studies have used the SDS to directly examine the efficacy of clozapine for primary negative symptoms. In a double-blind study, clozapine was observed to be effective for positive symptoms in both deficit and nondeficit patients. In contrast, only nondeficit patients exhibited a negative response to clozapine, with the response primarily limited to the SANS anhedonia/asociality subscale (Breier et al. 1994; Buchanan et al. 1998). The observed benefit was based on a slight improvement of the subscale items in the clozapine-treated patients and a mild worsening of the items in the haloperidol-treated patients. An important feature of this study—and a possible explanation of the limited negative symptom response observed in nondeficit patients—was the low baseline level of EPS. Similar results were observed in an open-labeled study conducted in inpatients with schizophrenia (Conley et al. 1997). Patients with the deficit form of schizophrenia shared with nondeficit patients the positive symptom advantage of clozapine, but deficit patients failed to exhibit any negative symptom benefit.

In combination, these studies suggest that clozapine's negative symptom efficacy is limited to secondary negative symptoms. The initial enthusiasm for clozapine as a treatment for negative symptoms was largely based on a failure to take into account its ability to ameliorate secondary causes of negative symptoms. Although this conclusion can be debated (Meltzer 1995), it is strongly supported by the results of recent double-blind studies, which have failed to document any comparative therapeutic advantage of clozapine over haloperidol for negative symptoms (Marder et al. 1997) or any independent effect of clozapine for negative symptoms after controlling for either EPS (Rosenheck et al. 1997) or positive symptoms (Rosenheck et al. 1999).

The clozapine experience suggests that assertions of superior negative symptom efficacy need to be carefully examined in the context of the methodological issues previously described. For example, risperidone has been pronounced to have superior efficacy for negative symptoms compared with conventional antipsychotics. This claim is primarily based on the results of the North American multicenter study (Chouinard et al. 1993; Marder and Meibach 1994). In that study, risperidone at 6 mg/day was more effective than placebo in alleviating negative symptoms, and there was a trend for risperidone to be more effective than haloperidol at 20 mg/day. However, in the European multicenter study (Peuskens 1995), there were no significant differences in negative symptom efficacy between risperidone at therapeutic doses (4 and 8 mg/day) and risperidone at 1 mg/day (used as a subtherapeutic control dose) or between the therapeutic risperidone doses and haloperidol at 10 mg/day. The loss of the presumed therapeutic advantage for negative symptoms when risperidone was compared with a lower therapeutic haloperidol dose raises serious questions about risperidone's purported superior efficacy for negative symptoms.

Approaches for Assessing Primary Negative Symptom Response

Several approaches have been developed for facilitating evaluation of the primary negative symptom efficacy of a drug. These approaches have principally been designed to address two methodological issues: the primary/secondary negative symptom distinction and the role of confounding variables. The most widely used approaches involve the use of statistical techniques to control for confounding variables. These techniques range from bivariate correlations to path analyses. The underlying assumption in these approaches is as follows: If the negative symptom variance attributable to changes in variables that cause secondary negative symptoms is removed, then the variance that remains reflects changes in primary negative symptoms.

The correlation between change in negative symptoms and change in other symptoms has been used to examine the effects of conventional antipsychotic withdrawal (Miller et al. 1994a), conventional antipsychotic treatment (Tandon et al. 1990, 1993b), and clozapine treatment on negative symptoms (Lieberman et al. 1994; Miller et al. 1994b; Tandon et al. 1993a). Multiple regression models have also been employed. Miller and colleagues (1994b) used this approach to examine the ability of positive, depressive, and extrapyramidal symptoms to predict end-of-study negative symptom scores after covarying for baseline negative symptom scores. One limitation of their application of these models is that because both primary and secondary negative symptoms contribute to the baseline negative symptom score, that score is not independent of the other symptom measures used in the analysis (Carpenter et al. 1995).

In post hoc analyses of the North American multicenter risperidone and the North American double-blind olanzapine studies, path analysis was used in an attempt to delineate the respective contributions of changes in secondary causes of negative symptoms (Möller et al. 1995; Tollefson and Sanger 1997). After the researchers corrected for changes in positive, affective, and/ or extrapyramidal symptoms, an additional significant "direct" effect on negative symptoms was observed for both risperidone and olanzapine that was not observed for haloperidol. However, unexplained variance is not necessarily equal to primary negative symptoms, for at least two reasons. First, as previously discussed, rating instruments have limited sensitivity and reliability, which restricts their ability to capture the full extent to which secondary causes of negative symptoms may be influencing the observed variability in the severity of negative symptoms. Second, the causes of secondary negative symptoms vary across individuals and extend beyond the symptom measures assessed in the study, which limits the ability to statistically control for all potential sources of secondary negative symptoms.

An alternative approach for evaluating primary negative symptom response is to select as subjects patients characterized by high levels of negative symptoms and low levels of other symptoms. This method has been used to assess the efficacy of amisulpiride, glycine, and d-cycloserine for negative symptoms (Boyer et al. 1995; Goff et al. 1995; Javitt et al. 1994; Paillere-Martinot et al. 1995). The rationale for this approach is that to the extent that secondary causes of negative symptoms are either absent or minimally present in the study population, the observed negative symptoms are more likely to represent primary negative symptoms. This approach may provide a reasonable estimate of primary negative symptom efficacy if potential sources of secondary negative symptoms are actually eliminated.

Recommendations

In light of the issues discussed here, we propose the following guidelines for the treatment of patients with negative symptoms and the following procedures for the design of clinical trials for the assessment of primary negative symptom response.

With respect to the treatment of the patient with negative symptoms, the most important issue is the differentiation of primary and secondary negative symptoms. Although there is currently no known available treatment for primary negative symptoms, a number of effective treatments are available for secondary negative symptoms (Buchanan et al. 1996). If a patient presents with negative symptoms, he or she should be evaluated for the presence of persistent positive, depressive, and/or anxious symptoms, and/or for EPS. If a patient presents with persistent positive symptoms, that patient should either have his or her medication dosage adjusted or be offered a clozapine trial. Similarly, if a patient presents with affective symptoms, he or she should be treated with adjunctive antidepressant or antianxiety agents. With a patient presents with negative symptoms and marked EPS, the clinician should reduce the antipsychotic dosage, initiate treatment with or increase the dosage of antiparkinsonian medication, or offer the patient a trial with an antipsychotic that is less likely to cause EPS (e.g., a new-generation antipsychotic). The clinician may use a modified version of either the SANS (i.e., minus the Inappropriate Affect, Poverty of Content of Speech, Impersistence at Work or School, Grooming and Hygiene, and Attention items) or the PANSS (i.e., minus the Difficulty in Abstract Thinking and Stereotyped Thinking items) to monitor negative symptom response to the intervention in question.

With regard to the design of clinical trials to assess primary negative symptom response, the most important step is to select patients with primary, enduring negative symptoms (i.e., patients with the deficit form of schizophrenia) for entry into the study. The a priori selection of these patients ensures that the patients enrolled in the clinical trial actually have the psychopathology of interest. At present, the SDS is the only available instrument specifically designed for this purpose. Nondeficit patients with secondary negative symptoms may also be included in the study sample. Including such patients allows evaluation of the experimental intervention's effect on secondary negative symptoms.

No currently available instruments are specifically designed to assess primary negative symptom change or to distinguish change in primary negative symptoms from change in secondary negative symptoms. The SANS or the PANSS, modified as described above, may be used to assess changes in negative symptoms during clinical trials. Other design refinements permit the assertion that observed negative symptom change involves primary negative symptoms. Such refinements include enrolling patients with primary negative symptoms and controlling for the influence of secondary causes of negative symptoms. The need to control for secondary negative symptoms persists despite the inclusion of deficit syndrome patients, because such patients may have either superimposed secondary negative symptoms or fluctuations in symptom intensity due to secondary causes.

There are several ways to control for the influence of secondary causes of negative symptoms. One approach is to select a clinically stable patient cohort with minimal levels of secondary sources of negative symptoms. Alternatively, one may select clinically stable patients, without consideration of the presence of other symptoms, and conduct concurrent assessments of potential causes of secondary negative symptoms, including positive, extrapyramidal, depressive, and anxiety symptoms. The concurrent assessments of other symptoms may then be used to statistically control for the influence of secondary sources of negative symptoms. Although this second approach ensures the availability of suitable patients, its validity is potentially undermined by the considerations discussed earlier in this chapter. A combination of these two approaches may provide the optimal design. Regardless of which strategy is employed, the use of clinically stable rather than acutely ill patients is of primary importance.

If these procedures are followed, a significant reduction of negative symptoms in patients with the deficit form of schizophrenia that cannot be accounted for by changes in secondary sources of negative symptoms would provide prima facie evidence for the efficacy of a drug for primary negative symptoms. In contrast, if significant negative symptom reductions were observed only in nondeficit patients, the negative symptom efficacy of the drug would be judged to be limited to secondary negative symptoms.

Summary

Several methodological issues are important in the evaluation of the therapeutic efficacy of a clinical intervention for negative symptoms. To the extent that these issues are addressed, our ability to validly assess the efficacy of these interventions will be significantly enhanced. The isolation of primary negative symptoms for assessments of treatment efficacy is an example of the general trend to single out specific symptom complexes or cognitive impairments for investigation. The methodological principles outlined for the assessment of negative symptom efficacy will also apply to the investigation of therapeutic efficacy in these other specific areas.

References

Andreasen NC: Negative symptoms in schizophrenia: definition and reliability. Arch Gen Psychiatry 39:784–788, 1982

Andreasen NC, Arndt S, Alliger R, et al: Symptoms of schizophrenia. Arch Gen Psychiatry 52:341–351, 1995

Beasley CM, Tollefson G, Tran P, et al: Olanzapine versus placebo and haloperidol. Neuropsychopharmacology 14:111–123, 1996

Berrios GE: Positive and negative symptoms and Jackson: a conceptual history. Arch Gen Psychiatry 42:95–97, 1985

Boyer P, Lecrubier Y, Peuch J, et al: Treatment of negative symptoms in schizophrenia with amisulpride. Br J Psychiatry 166:68–72, 1995

Breier A, Schreiber JL, Dyer J, et al: National Institute of Mental Health longitudinal study of chronic schizophrenia: prognosis and predictors of outcome. Arch Gen Psychiatry 48:239–246, 1991

Breier A, Buchanan RW, Kirkpatrick B, et al: Effects of clozapine on positive and negative symptoms in outpatients with schizophrenia. Am J Psychiatry 151:20–26, 1994

Buchanan RW, Carpenter WT Jr: Domains of psychopathology and approach to the reduction of heterogeneity in schizophrenia. J Nerv Ment Dis 182:193–204, 1994

Buchanan RW, Gold JM: Negative symptoms: diagnosis, treatment and prognosis. Int Clin Psychopharmacol 11 (suppl 2):3–11, 1996

Buchanan RW, Strauss ME, Kirkpatrick B, et al: Neuropsychological impairments in deficit vs. nondeficit forms of schizophrenia. Arch Gen Psychiatry 51:804–812, 1994

Buchanan RW, Brandes M, Breier A: Pharmacological strategies for treating negative symptoms, in The New Pharmacotherapy of Schizophrenia. Edited by Breier A. Washington, DC, American Psychiatric Association, 1996, pp 179–204

Buchanan RW, Strauss ME, Breier A, et al: Attentional impairments in deficit and nondeficit forms of schizophrenia. Am J Psychiatry 154:363–370, 1997

Bustillo JR, Thaker G, Buchanan RW, et al: Visual information-processing impairments in deficit and nondeficit schizophrenia. Am J Psychiatry 154:647–754, 1997

Carpenter WT Jr: The treatment of negative symptoms: pharmacological and methodological issues. Br J Psychiatry 168:17–22, 1996

Carpenter WT Jr, Heinrichs DW, Alphs LD: Treatment of negative symptoms. Schizophr Bull 11:440–452, 1985

Carpenter WT Jr, Heinrichs DW, Wagman AMI: Deficit and nondeficit forms of schizophrenia: the concept. Am J Psychiatry 145:578–583, 1988

Carpenter WT Jr, Buchanan RW, Kirkpatrick B, et al: Strong inference, theory falsification, and the neuroanatomy of schizophrenia. Arch Gen Psychiatry 50:825–831, 1993

Carpenter WT Jr, Conley RR, Buchanan RW, et al: Patient response and resource management: another view of clozapine treatment of schizophrenia. Am J Psychiatry 152:827–832, 1995

Chouinard G, Jones B, Remington G, et al: A Canadian multicenter placebo-controlled study of fixed doses of risperidone and haloperidol in the treatment of chronic schizophrenic patients. J Clin Psychopharmacol 13:25–40, 1993

Conley R, Richardson C, Tamminga C: Treatment of primary negative symptoms (abstract). Biol Psychiatry 42 (1 suppl):204S, 1997

Dworkin RH, Lenzenweger MF, Moldin SO, et al: A multidimensional approach to the genetics of schizophrenia. Am J Psychiatry 145:1077–1083, 1988

Fenton WS, McGlashan TH: Testing systems for assessment of negative symptoms in schizophrenia. Arch Gen Psychiatry 49:179–184, 1992

Glovinsky D, Kirch DG, Wyatt RJ: Early antipsychotic response to resumption of neuroleptics in drug-free chronic schizophrenic patients. Biol Psychiatry 31:968–970, 1992

Goff DC, Tsai G, Manoach DS, et al: Dose-finding trial of D-cycloserine added to neuroleptics for negative symptoms in schizophrenia. Am J Psychiatry 152:1213–1215, 1995

Goff DC, Tsai G, Levitt J, et al: A placebo-controlled trial of D-cycloserine added to conventional neuroleptics in patients with schizophrenia. Arch Gen Psychiatry 56:21–27, 1999

Goldberg SC: Negative and deficit symptoms in schizophrenia do respond to neuroleptics. Schizophr Bull 11:453–456, 1985

Green MF: What are the functional consequences of neurocognitive deficits in schizophrenia? Am J Psychiatry 153:321–330, 1996

Heinrichs DW, Hanlon TE, Carpenter WT Jr: The Quality of Life Scale: an instrument for rating the schizophrenic deficit syndrome. Schizophr Bull 10:388–398, 1984

Heresco-Levy U, Javitt DC, Ermilov M, et al: Double-blind, placebo-controlled, crossover trial of glycine adjuvant therapy for treatment-resistant schizophrenia. Br J Psychiatry 169:610–617, 1996

Heresco-Levy U, Javitt DC, Ermilov M, et al: Efficacy of high-dose glycine in the treatment of enduring negative symptoms of schizophrenia. Arch Gen Psychiatry 56:29–36, 1999

Javitt DC, Zylberman I, Zukin SR, et al: Amelioration of negative symptoms in schizophrenia by glycine. Am J Psychiatry 151:1234–1236, 1994

Kane J, Honigfeld G, Singer J, et al: Clozapine for the treatment-resistant schizophrenic: a double-blind comparison with chlorpromazine. Arch Gen Psychiatry 45:789–796, 1988

Kay SR, Sevy S: Pyramidical model of schizophrenia. Schizophr Bull 16:537–544, 1990

Kay SR, Fiszbein A, Opler LA: The Positive and Negative Syndrome Scale (PANSS) for schizophrenia. Schizophr Bull 13:261–276, 1987

Kendler KS, Gruenberg AM, Tsuang MT: A DSM-III family study of the nonschizophrenic psychotic disorders. Am J Psychiatry 143:1098–1105, 1986

Kirkpatrick B, Buchanan RW: The neural basis of the deficit syndrome of schizophrenia. J Nerv Ment Dis 178:545–555, 1990

Kirkpatrick B, Buchanan RW, McKenney PD, et al: The Schedule for the Deficit Syndrome: an instrument for research in schizophrenia. Psychiatry Res 30:119–123, 1989

Kirkpatrick B, Ram R, Amador XF, et al: Summer birth and the deficit syndrome of schizophrenia. Am J Psychiatry 155:1221–1226, 1998

Kraepelin E: Dementia Praecox and Paraphrenia (1919). Translated by Barclay RM. Huntingdon, NY, RE Krieger, 1971

Liddle PF, Friston KJ, Frith CD, et al: Patterns of cerebral blood flow in schizophrenia. Br J Psychiatry 160:179–186, 1992

Lieberman JA, Safferman AZ, Pollack S, et al: Clinical effects of clozapine in chronic schizophrenia: response to treatment and predictors of outcome. Am J Psychiatry 151:1744–1752, 1994

Leiderman E, Zylberman I, Zukin SR, et al: Preliminary investigation of high-dose oral glycine on serum levels and negative symptoms in schizophrenia: an open label trial. Biol Psychiatry 39:213–215, 1996

Lukoff D, Nuechterlein KH, Ventura J: Symptom monitoring in the rehabilitation of schizophrenic patients. [See Appendix A: Manual for expanded Brief Psychiatric Rating Scale (BPRS).] Schizophr Bull 12:578–602, 1986

Marder SR, Meibach RC: Risperidone in the treatment of schizophrenia. Am J Psychiatry 151:825–835, 1994

Marder SR, Kane JM, Schooler NR, et al: Effectiveness of clozapine in treatment resistant schizophrenia (abstract). Schizophr Res 24:187, 1997

Meltzer HY: Clozapine: pattern of efficacy in treatment-resistant schizophrenia, in Novel Antipsychotic Drugs. Edited by Meltzer HY. New York, Raven, 1992, pp 33–46

Meltzer HY: Clozapine: is another view valid? (editorial). Am J Psychiatry 15:821–825, 1995

Miller DD, Flaum M, Arndt S, et al: Effect of antipsychotic withdrawal on negative symptoms in schizophrenia. Neuropsychopharmacology 11:11–20, 1994a

Miller DD, Perry PJ, Cadoret RJ, et al: Clozapine's effect on negative symptoms in treatment-refractory schizophrenics. Compr Psychiatry 35:8–15, 1994b

Möller H-J, Muller H, Borison RL, et al: A path-analytical approach to differentiate between direct and indirect drug effects on negative symptoms in schizophrenic patients: a re-evaluation of the North American risperidone study. Eur Arch Psychiatry Clin Neurosci 245:45–49, 1995

Paillere-Martinot M-L, Lecrubier Y, Martinot J-L, et al: Improvement of some schizophrenic deficit symptoms with low doses of amisulpride. Am J Psychiatry 152:130–133, 1995

Peuskens J: Risperidone in the treatment of patients with chronic schizophrenia: a multi-national, multi-centre, double-blind, parallel-group study versus haloperidol. Risperidone Study Group. Br J Psychiatry 166:712–726, 1995

Pickar D, Owen RR, Litman RE, et al: Clinical and biologic response to clozapine in patients with schizophrenia: crossover comparison with fluphenazine. Arch Gen Psychiatry 49:345–353, 1992

Rosenheck R, Charney D, Cramer J, et al: A randomized, double-blind trial of the efficacy and cost-effectiveness of clozapine (abstract). Schizophr Res 24:188, 1997

Rosenheck R, Dunn L, Peszke M, et al: Impact of clozapine on negative symptoms and on the deficit syndrome in refractory schizophrenia. Am J Psychiatry 156:88–93, 1999

Sommers AA: "Negative symptoms": conceptual and methodological problems. Schizophr Bull 11:364–379, 1985

Strauss ME: Relations of symptoms to cognitive deficits in schizophrenia. Schizophr Bull 19:215–231, 1993

Tandon R, Goldman RS, Goodson J, et al: Mutability and relationship between positive and negative symptoms during neuroleptic treatment in schizophrenia. Biol Psychiatry 27:1323–1326, 1990

Tandon R, Goldman R, DeQuardo JR, et al: Positive and negative symptoms covary during clozapine treatment in schizophrenia. J Psychiatr Res 27:341–347, 1993a

Tandon R, Ribeiro SCM, DeQuardo JR, et al: Covariance of positive and negative symptoms during neuroleptic treatment in schizophrenia: a replication. Biol Psychiatry 34:495–497, 1993b

Tollefson GD, Sanger TM: Negative symptoms: a path analytic approach to a double-blind, placebo- and haloperidol-controlled clinical trial with olanzapine. Am J Psychiatry 154:466–474, 1997

Tsai G, Yang P, Chung L-C, et al: D-serine added to antipsychotics for the treatment of schizophrenia. Biol Psychiatry 44:1081–1089, 1998

Waltrip RW, Buchanan RW, Carpenter WT Jr, et al: Borna disease virus antibodies and the deficit syndrome of schizophrenia. Schizophr Res 23:253–257, 1997

Wing JK, Brown GW: Institutionalism and Schizophrenia. A Comparative Study of Three Mental Hospitals. Cambridge, UK, Cambridge University Press, 1970

Issues in the Assessment of Negative Symptom Treatment Response

Peg Nopoulos, M.D.
Del D. Miller, Pharm.D., M.D.
Michael Flaum, M.D.
Nancy C. Andreasen, M.D., Ph.D.

The question of whether the traditional or the new neuroleptics have a greater impact on negative symptoms has elicited considerable interest during the past few years. As investigators have examined strategies for measuring the efficacy of new neuroleptics for negative symptoms more critically, a number of problems have been noted. Several factors are important to consider in the assessment of negative symptoms and their response to treatment. Two basic issues are 1) ensuring the validity of negative symptom assessment (cross-sectionally and over time) and 2) distinguishing whether drugs are having an impact on primary negative or secondary negative symptoms. In this chapter we first address the issue of validity of negative symptom assessment. We then review the advantages and disadvantages of a variety of strategies aimed at elucidating the primary versus secondary distinction.

This research was supported in part by National Institute of Mental Health Grants MH31,593, MH40856, and MHCRC43271; a Research Scientist Award (MHOO625) to Dr. Andreasen; and an Established Investigator Award to Dr. Andreasen from the National Alliance for Research on Schizophrenia and Depression.

Validity of Negative Symptom Assessment

Although much emphasis has been placed on the importance of the primary negative versus secondary negative distinction, the more global question of the general validity of negative symptom assessment is rarely addressed. The entire notion of distinguishing between primary and secondary negative symptoms may be a moot point if the ways in which negative symptoms are assessed are not valid. The development of diagnostic instruments and rating scales has been of great utility in psychiatric research for quantifying psychiatric signs and symptoms. Regardless of the instrument used, the information it elicits is only as reliable as its source. However, many factors may interfere with a schizophrenia patient's ability to accurately report his or her symptoms. The validity of negative symptom assessment needs to be considered, especially given that much of the information reflected in the data obtained from instrument ratings is based directly on patient self-report.

Our group recently reported a study designed to evaluate how accurately patients with psychotic disorders could describe their symptoms (Flaum et al. 1993). Fifty-five subjects with psychotic disorders were evaluated with a semistructured interview, the Comprehensive Assessment of Symptoms and History (CASH; Andreasen et al. 1992), which includes the Scale for the Assessment of Negative Symptoms (SANS; Andreasen 1989) and the Scale for the Assessment of Positive Symptoms (SAPS; Andreasen 1984). One interviewer assigned ratings solely on the basis of information provided by the patient. A second interviewer based ratings on information obtained from a "best informant"; this individual was usually the patient's mother. Finally, a consensus set of ratings was established based on review of several sources: inpatient evaluation, medical records, and information from the patient, family, and mental health care professionals who help care for the patient.

Paired *t* tests were used to compare proband, informant, and consensus ratings for the five global negative ratings from the SANS: anhedonia/asociality, avolition/apathy, affective flattening, alogia, and attentional impairment. The comparisons showed that there were wide discrepancies in ratings among the three sources of information. The proband-based ratings of severity for negative symptoms were all significantly lower than the consensus ratings; however, there were no differences between informant ratings and the consensus ratings for any of the negative symptoms. Thus, the ratings based on information from family members closely approximated the consensus or "gold standard" ratings, whereas patients themselves consistently underrated the severity of their negative symptoms. These findings suggest that structured interviews that are based on subjects' own responses may be quite inaccurate in measuring negative symptoms. This conclusion may be particularly important for assessment of treatment response, because underestimation of a subject's negative symptoms at intake into a study will certainly blunt or even mask any improvement seen over time. Therefore, information about negative symptoms may be most valid when obtained from an informant other than, or in addition to, the patient.

This problem of underrating of negative symptoms by patients is exemplified in the following case vignette.

> Mr. C is a 27-year-old man with schizophrenia who lives at home with his mother. Until his early 20s, he was functioning quite well: he was able to attend and complete 2 years of college before he became ill. He is somewhat embarrassed and resentful that he now lives with his parents and relies on their help. When asked by the physician if he is socially active, Mr. C states that he is, and that he and his friends go out at least once a week. He also states that he is not sedentary, is up early in the morning, grooms himself, and spends his days helping his mother around the house.
>
> Mr. C's mother, however, tells a very different story. She reports that Mr. C has been abandoned by all of the friends he used to see and that he has not been "out" to socialize in several months. Furthermore, she states that his daily routine is to sleep for 12–15 hours and, on waking, to lie on the couch watching television for the remainder of the day. Rarely does Mr. C help around the house, and his mother has to remind him frequently to shower and groom himself.

This example highlights the importance of obtaining information from family members to corroborate patients' self-reports.

The Primary Versus Secondary Distinction

Originally introduced by Bleuler (1911/1950), the primary versus secondary distinction has more recently been articulated and emphasized by Carpenter et al. (1988). Bleuler was attempting to identify the symptoms of schizophrenia that he regarded as most fundamental: those that could explain all other related symptoms. From Bleuler's point of view, the most basic or primary symptoms were those involving cognition and emotion (i.e., associations, affect, ambivalence, autism, attention, avolition). He regarded delusions and hallucinations as secondary to these more primary cognitive and emotional symptoms and as nonspecific to schizophrenia. Carpenter and colleagues have supplemented this psychological and clinical perspective with their concept of the *deficit syndrome* (Buchanan et al. 1990; Carpenter et al. 1988; Heinrichs et al. 1984; Kirkpatrick et al. 1989). This syndrome is characterized by the presence of negative symptoms that are "enduring," in the sense that they cannot be explained by any of a variety of possible confounders, such as extrapyramidal side effects (EPS), depression, positive symptoms, and inadequate social stimulation. Carpenter and colleagues have argued that in order to identify primary or enduring negative symptoms, these various confounders must be ruled out as causes through a careful clinical assessment.

While Carpenter and colleagues' emphasis on distinguishing primary from secondary negative symptoms has been useful and important, clinicians and investigators have often failed to recognize that positive symptoms may also be secondary. A number of conditions can produce secondary positive symptoms, and these should (at least theoretically) be ruled out in any careful pharmacological or neurobiological study of positive symptoms. Just as drugs can produce EPS (e.g., akinesia) and thereby mimic negative symptoms, so, too, can drugs produce akathisia and thereby mimic the agitation and disorganized behavior that we associate with positive symptoms. Just as depression can mimic negative symptoms, so, too, can euphoria and grandiosity mimic positive symptoms such as grandiose paranoia. Negative symptoms can also produce positive symptoms; for example, severe avolition can lead to disorganized behavior. If one considers attentional impairment to be a negative symptom, then it, too, can be seen as leading to a wide variety of positive symptoms, ranging from disorganized speech and behavior to hallucinations.

The major problem with the primary versus secondary distinction is the complexity and diversity of schizophrenia. Although these distinctions make sense on some levels, in real life it is difficult to obtain pure measures. In real life, symptoms co-occur much of the time.

Nonetheless, the development of new antipsychotics, some of which may have the potential to treat negative as well as positive symptoms, has led to an interest in attempting to distinguish both between positive and negative symptoms and between primary and secondary negative symptoms.

Strategies for Disentangling Primary and Secondary Negative Symptoms

Several different strategies are available with which to disentangle primary and secondary negative symptoms in clinical drug trials. These include

1) targeting sample selection to a more "primary" group, 2) using shorter versus longer drug washouts, 3) using a sample of "deficit syndrome" patients, 4) using clinical decision-making to distinguish primary from secondary negative symptoms, and 5) using statistical techniques. Efforts by pharmaceutical companies to determine whether new therapeutic agents are efficacious for the treatment of negative symptoms can use one of several different strategies. Each of these strategies has specific strengths and weaknesses, and none will resolve the problem completely.

Selection of More "Primary" Samples

One strategy for examining the effects of new antipsychotic medications is to identify an informative group of patients low in potential confounding factors in whom efficacy can be tested. Under this strategy, the investigator attempts to select a group that is prima facie characterized by primary negative symptoms. One example of such a group is patients who rate high on negative symptoms and low on positive symptoms. These patients are then selected to have both an abundance of the symptoms whose response will be evaluated (primary negative symptoms) and very few of the symptoms that may confound the assessment of improvement (positive symptoms). Although this strategy is ideal, it may be difficult to apply in reality. First, patients who meet these initial entry criteria are relatively difficult to find. The most serious problem that may arise is a change in the clinical picture as a consequence of the placebo lead-in phase in clinical drug trials. Emergence of positive symptoms or depression, as well as diminution in EPS, during this time period could change inferences about the underlying nature of negative symptoms.

Shorter Versus Longer Drug Washouts

Placebo lead-in phases are standard in most clinical drug trials. Their rationale is to establish a "baseline" against which patients' functioning with the new agent can be compared. Placebo lead-in periods vary from a few days to a few weeks. Shorter periods are usually selected for convenience, but these are likely to be much less successful in establishing a true baseline. During brief lead-in periods (e.g., 3–5 days), little change in clinical symptoms of any type is seen. On the other hand, longer periods of drug withdrawal (e.g., 3 weeks) are typically characterized by an emergence of positive symptoms and a decrease in EPS. A study conducted in our laboratory (Miller et al. 1994) to investigate the effects of antipsychotic withdrawal in 59 patients over a 3-week period demonstrated significant increases in both negative symptoms and disorganization symptoms, as well as a decrease in EPS, as rated by the SANS (Andreasen 1989), the SAPS (Andreasen 1984), and the Simpson-Angus scale (Simpson and Angus 1970). During this 3-week period, no changes were seen in psychotic symptoms or in depressive symptoms as measured by the Hamilton Depression Scale (Hamilton 1960). Drug washouts lasting 3 weeks or longer provide a truer baseline than do shorter washouts. However, it was difficult to determine whether the increasing severity of negative symptoms in these patients was secondary to the change in positive symptoms or the change in EPS. When we examined correlational relationships, we found that the negative symptom increase correlated with increasing disorganization and psychoticism, but not with decreasing EPS. Such correlational analyses do not permit directional inferences, however, and thus we could not definitively determine whether the increasing disorganization caused the increased negative symptoms or vice versa.

Selection of "Deficit Syndrome" Samples

In the short–placebo lead-in strategy, the two domains of psychopathology (negative and positive) are used as continuous variables that can then be separated by identifying extreme groups of a heterogeneous population (high negative symptoms, low positive symptoms). Given that positive and negative symptoms of schizophrenia have been found to be independent domains, this strategy could be taken one step further by identifying a group of patients who are considered to be a more homogeneous and possibly etiologically distinct group of patients—those who suffer from the deficit syndrome (as defined by Carpenter and his group). Such patients are identified through a careful and systematic assessment based on retrospective longitudinal observation. Carpenter et al. (1988; Kirkpatrick et al. 1989) have developed a structured assessment instrument (the Schedule for the Deficit Syndrome [SDS]) and operational criteria for identifying the deficit syndrome. According to these criteria, subjects must display prominent negative symptoms for at least 12 months in the absence of likely secondary causes. Carpenter and colleagues have demonstrated adequate reliability for these assessment tools and have used them within their center to categorize patients as having the deficit versus the nondeficit form of schizophrenia.

What is the difference between a sample of patients characterized by mostly primary negative symptoms (as discussed above) and a sample of patients with the deficit syndrome? These two groups appear to have a large amount of overlap in their definitions. One explanation is continuum-based and suggests that deficit patients should be considered extreme cases of the mostly "primary" negative group. On the other hand, Carpenter's group has supported the notion that the deficit syndrome is etiologically distinct from other "types" of schizophrenia and therefore should not be considered as just an extreme expression of primary negative symptoms. They and others have published a series of reports in which the validity of the deficit versus nondeficit distinction has been supported by differences in a variety of areas, including cognitive function (Buchanan et al. 1994), magnetic resonance imaging (MRI) measures (Buchanan et al. 1993), risk for spontaneous dyskinesia (Fenton et al. 1994), eye movement abnormalities (Ross et al. 1996), Borna disease virus seropositivity (Waltrip et al. 1997) and course and outcome (Fenton and McGlashan 1994).

Regardless of whether deficit syndrome patients constitute the extreme end of a "primary negative" group or a separate group with distinct etiology, it has been proposed that it may be helpful to include these patients in clinical trials that attempt to determine whether negative symptoms respond to treatment. The rationale for this strategy is that the potential underlying causes of secondary negative symptoms have already been ruled out. If deficit patients show an improvement in negative symptoms with the new therapeutic agent, their response can be interpreted as a demonstration of the agent's effect on primary negative symptoms. Although this strategy has much to commend it, it also involves potential problems. Cross-center reliability in the assessment of the deficit syndrome is not yet well established, which would make this approach more difficult to apply in multicenter trials. Also, patients who fulfill criteria for the deficit syndrome represent only a minority of patients with schizophrenia. Carpenter and colleagues have estimated that only 20%–30% of schizophrenia patients have the deficit syndrome, and others have suggested that the incidence of deficit syndrome in first-episode patients is actually much smaller (Mayerhoff et al. 1994). Although deficit syndrome patients are considered to represent a homogeneous group, limiting a study sample to these patients would invariably result in the practical problem of low numbers of subjects, especially if the patients are first-episode patients. Furthermore, because of the longitudinal perspective of the deficit syndrome criteria, their application may lead to changing conclusions.

Clinical Decision-Making

Although the strategy of selecting deficit syndrome samples may be considered the "gold standard" by virtue of providing the most homogeneous and purest form of the target symptoms, it may not be practical in a clinical setting. The question then becomes whether clinicians can reliably distinguish between primary and secondary symptoms in the absence of extensive longitudinal information or highly specialized rating scales and training methods. Our group was able to address this question in the context of the DSM-IV (American Psychiatric Association 1994) schizophrenia field trial project (Flaum and Andreasen 1995). The reliability of the primary versus secondary distinction was examined in a multicenter sample of 462 subjects with nonorganic psychotic disorders. Each subject was assessed by two raters. An interrater design (i.e., conjoint interviews) was used with half of the subjects and a test–retest design (i.e., independent interviews by two raters conducted 1 day apart), with the other half. All raters used the same semistructured interview instrument, which included an abbreviated version of the SANS. In addition to the usual SANS ratings, raters were asked to indicate whether, in their opinion, the symptom in question was primary, secondary, or unknown (inadequate information to assess). No formal training was provided.

For the sample as a whole, each of the negative symptoms was judged to be primary about twice as often as secondary. This ratio varied substantially across diagnoses. For subjects assigned a DSM-III-R (American Psychiatric Association 1987) diagnosis of schizophrenia ($n = 240$), the primary:secondary ratio was consistently around 4:1 (Figure 2–1). For all other patients (including those assigned a diagnosis of psychotic mood disorder, schizoaffective disorder, delusional disorder, and other psychotic disorders), the ratio of primary to secondary negative symptoms was approximately 1:1. For each of the negative symptoms, raters indicated that they had adequate information to make the primary versus secondary distinction more than 90% of the time.

Table 2–1 shows the interrater and the test–retest reliability of the primary versus secondary distinctions made by pairs of raters who had agreed that the negative symptom was present. Kappa values for interrater reliability ranged from 0.48 to 0.68 (median = 0.50). Kappas for test–retest reliability ranged from 0.34 to 0.66 (median = 0.38). Therefore, despite raters' indications that adequate information existed with which to distinguish between the two types of negative symptoms, the interrater and test–retest reliabilities of making the distinctions were marginal to poor. These findings suggest that clinical decision-making may not be the best method for disentangling primary from secondary negative symptoms and call into question the usefulness of this type of assessment.

One possible way to increase the reliability with which the primary versus secondary distinction can be made is to assess the symptoms after employing pharmacological interventions geared to remove confounders. Take,

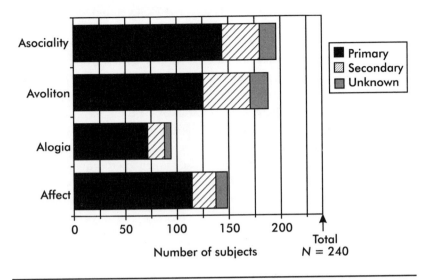

FIGURE 2–1. Frequency of primary and secondary negative symptoms among patients with a DSM-III-R diagnosis of schizophrenia.

Source. Reprinted from Flaum M, Andreasen NC: "The Reliability of Distinguishing Primary Versus Secondary Negative Symptoms." *Comprehensive Psychiatry* 36:421–427, 1995. Copyright © 1995, W. B. Saunders Co. Used with permission.

TABLE 2–1. Reliability of distinguishing primary and secondary negative symptoms

Negative symptom	Interrater reliability kappa (*n*)	Test–retest reliability kappa (*n*)
Affective flattening	0.685 (85)	0.368 (74)
Alogia	0.482 (54)	0.659 (45)
Avolition/apathy	0.483 (91)	0.400 (112)
Asociality/anhedonia	0.512 (104)	0.339 (127)

Note. These reliability coefficients refer only to the reliability of making the primary versus secondary distinction, rather than also reflecting the reliability of assessing the presence or severity of negative symptoms. They are based on pairs of raters who 1) agreed that the negative symptom was present to at least a mild degree, and 2) both indicated that adequate information was available to make the primary versus secondary distinction.

Source. Reprinted from Flaum M, Andreasen NC: "The Reliability of Distinguishing Primary Versus Secondary Negative Symptoms." *Comprehensive Psychiatry* 36:421–427, 1995. Copyright © 1995, W. B. Saunders Co. Used with permission.

for example, a patient who is akinetic. Lowering antipsychotic dosages or adding/increasing antiparkinsonian medications may improve or clear the akinesia, and one may then be able to determine that the negative symptoms were indeed secondary to medication side effects. However, this scenario is probably overly simplistic. It is improbable that a patient's symptom presentation would constitute a simple dichotomy (either primary or secondary negative symptoms); rather, there would most likely be components of each. In many cases, using pharmacological interventions in the attempt to distinguish between primary and secondary symptoms may only confound an already complex issue. Another downside to the use of such interventions is that the assessment cannot be made until the pharmacological intervention has been completed. Such a delay may be impractical for study protocols that require regular assessments.

Applying Statistical Techniques

Statistical techniques require 1) careful selection of rating instruments to evaluate each potential confounder and 2) use of analysis of variance (ANOVA) to separate out the sources of variance. For example, the application of ANOVA would require the use of repeated measures (typically on a weekly basis) to assess the various potential causes of secondary negative symptoms, such as EPS, depression, and positive symptoms. If—in response to treatment with a new therapeutic agent—patients show a significant improvement in negative symptoms over a 6- to 8-week period, ANOVA can be employed to determine whether the improvement in negative symptoms is statistically independent from changes in other symptoms. Obviously, if a new therapeutic agent is useful for treating schizophrenia, it is also likely to produce an improvement in positive (psychotic) symptoms. Such changes can be entered as a covariate in analyses to determine how much of the change in negative symptoms can be accounted for by concomitant changes in EPS, positive symptoms, and depressive symptoms. Statistical corrections of this type can be very helpful, but they are not definitive. They do not permit any assessment of directionality (i.e., whether an improvement in negative symptoms in conjunction with improvement in positive symptoms is secondary to the change in positive symptoms). Furthermore, such analyses do not allow any inferences about underlying neurochemical or biological mechanisms. Finally, statistical techniques typically require the use of multiple covariates. Many different factors could account for a change in negative symptoms, and when these factors are concurrent, it is difficult to determine clearly which of the various covariates may actually be having any observed effect.

Another useful statistical strategy is path analysis. This method, like ANOVA, attempts to determine whether the effect for negative symptoms is due to direct and/or indirect therapeutic action. Used in a study evaluating the effects of negative symptoms in a double-blind, placebo- and haloperidol-controlled trial with olanzapine (Tollefson and Sanger 1997), the path analytic strategy allowed for quantification of the various effects that could lead to negative symptom improvement. The *direct effect* is defined as the treatment effect remaining after covarying for improvement in other factors that could cause secondary negative symptoms, such as positive symptoms, depression, and drug side effects, which are the *indirect effects*. With use of this strategy, the drug's total effect on negative symptoms can be separated into the percentage due to direct effects and the percentage due to indirect effects.

For instance, in the Tollefson and Sanger study, patients in the olanzapine group showed a significantly greater improvement in negative symptoms compared with those in the placebo group. This result was then broken down, with path analysis, to show that olanzapine's direct effect on negative symptoms accounted for 55% of its advantage over placebo. In addition, the drug's indirect effect on negative symptoms via improvement of positive symptoms accounted for 43% of its advantage over placebo. The indirect effects on negative symptoms via improvement of depressive symptoms and EPS were much less significant, accounting for 5% and 3%, respectively, of olanzapine's advantage over placebo.

Summary and Conclusions

It may be helpful to step back and identify the various rationales for distinguishing between primary and secondary negative symptoms. There appear to be three main reasons for differentiating between these types of symptoms: a research rationale, a clinical drug trial rationale, and a clinical practice rationale. The research rationale aims at discovering the neurobiological mechanisms underlying negative symptoms. If the goal is to elucidate the neural substrates of negative symptoms, one strategy would be to identify the purest possible group, and this may indeed be Carpenter's deficit group. A sample of this type may be much more informative than one in which the negative symptoms are identified primarily through multivariate statistical techniques. If the goal is simply to study neurobiology, the problems of placebo lead-ins for clinical drug trials would probably not be relevant.

A second reason for distinguishing primary from secondary negative symptoms is to determine efficacy in clinical drug trials. For this objective, the main purpose is to avoid inferring that the specific symptom reduction has occurred, when in fact the mechanism has been side-effect reduction. In other words, many of the newer atypical neuroleptics produce fewer EPS. Critics have argued that the apparent efficacy of the newer medications for negative symptoms is simply a consequence of their reduced propensity to cause EPS, particularly in comparison with a drug such as haloperidol. It is in this context that either the application of statistical analyses with multivariate techniques or the selection of informative samples with relatively "pure" negative symptoms has been proposed. Although the informative-sample strategy may be preferable, the use of multivariate techniques may be adequate in some contexts. It is probably impossible to design a perfect clinical trial that will isolate the effects of medication on primary or negative symptoms. However, the next-best alternative is to design comparisons of typical and atypical neuroleptics that minimize as much as possible the confounding variables.

The third rationale for distinguishing primary from secondary negative symptoms is based on clinical practice. It is important that we conclude by considering this issue from the patient's point of view. The majority of patients feel more comfortable on the newer medications, largely as a consequence of their fewer side effects. We as pharmacologists and academicians would do well to remember that patients ultimately do not care whether their symptoms are primary or secondary. They care only about the fact that they feel better.

References

American Psychiatric Association: Diagnostic and Statistical Manual of Mental Disorders, 3rd Edition, Revised. Washington, DC, American Psychiatric Association, 1987

American Psychiatric Association: Diagnostic and Statistical Manual of Mental Disorders, 4th Edition. Washington, DC, American Psychiatric Association, 1994

Andreasen NC: The Scale for the Assessment of Positive Symptoms (SAPS). Iowa City, University of Iowa, 1984

Andreasen NC: The Scale for the Assessment of Negative Symptoms (SANS): conceptual and theoretical foundations. Br J Psychiatry 155 (suppl 7):49–58, 1989

Andreasen NC, Flaum M, Arndt S: The Comprehensive Assessment of Symptoms and History (CASH): an instrument for assessing psychopathology and diagnosis. Arch Gen Psychiatry 49:615–623, 1992

Bleuler E: Dementia Praecox or the Group of Schizophrenias (1911). Translated by Zinkin J. New York, International Universities Press, 1950

Buchanan RW, Kirkpatrick B, Heinrichs DW, et al: Clinical correlates of the deficit syndrome of schizophrenia. Am J Psychiatry 147:290–294, 1990

Buchanan RW, Breier A, Kirkpatrick B, et al: Structural abnormalities in deficit and nondeficit schizophrenia. Am J Psychiatry 150:59–65, 1993

Buchanan RW, Strauss ME, Kirkpatrick B, et al: Neuropsychological impairments in deficit vs nondeficit forms of schizophrenia. Arch Gen Psychiatry 51:804–811, 1994

Carpenter WT Jr, Heinrichs DW, Wagman AMI: Deficit and nondeficit forms of schizophrenia: the concept. Am J Psychiatry 145:578–583, 1988

Fenton WS, McGlashan TH: Antecedents, symptom progression, and long-term outcome of the deficit syndrome in schizophrenia. Am J Psychiatry 151:351–356, 1994

Fenton WS, Wyatt RJ, McGlashan TH: Risk factors for spontaneous dyskinesia in schizophrenia. Arch Gen Psychiatry 51:643–650, 1994

Flaum M, Andreasen NC: The reliability of distinguishing primary versus secondary negative symptoms. Compr Psychiatry 36:421–427, 1995

Flaum M, Hubbard WH, Arndt SV, et al: The validity of subjective reporting of positive and negative symptoms in schizophrenia (abstract). Schizophr Res 9:99, 1993

Hamilton M: A rating scale for depression. Journal of Psychiatry, Neurology, and Neurosurgery 23:56, 1960

Heinrichs DW, Hanlon TE, Carpenter WT Jr: The Quality of Life Scale: an instrument for rating the schizophrenic deficit syndrome. Schizophr Bull 10:388–398, 1984

Kirkpatrick B, Buchanan RW, McKenney PD, et al: The Schedule for the Deficit Syndrome: an instrument for research in schizophrenia. Psychiatry Res 30:119–123, 1989

Mayerhoff D, Loebel A, Alvir J, et al: The deficit state in first-episode schizophrenia. Am J Psychiatry 151:1417–1422, 1994

Miller DD, Flaum M, Arndt S, et al: Effect of antipsychotic withdrawal on negative symptoms in schizophrenia. Neuropsychopharmacology 11:11–20, 1994

Ross D, Thaker G, Buchanan R, et al: Association of abnormal smooth pursuit eye movements with the deficit syndrome in schizophrenic patients. Am J Psychiatry 153:1158–1165, 1 996

Simpson GM, Angus JWS: A rating scale for extrapyramidal side effects. Acta Psychiatr Scand Suppl 212:11–19, 1970

Tollefson GD, Sanger TM: Negative symptoms: a path analytic approach to a double-blind, placebo- and haloperidol-controlled clinical trial with olanzapine. Am J Psychiatry 154:466–474, 1997

Waltrip RW, Buchanan RW, Carpenter WT Jr, et al: Borna disease virus antibodies and the deficit syndrome of schizophrenia. Schizophr Res 23:253–258, 1997

3

Social Functioning and Its Relationship to Cognitive Deficits Over the Course of Schizophrenia

Susan L. Trumbetta, Ph.D.

Kim T. Mueser, Ph.D.

Mr. D is a 45-year-old man diagnosed with paranoid schizophrenia whose illness developed during his second year of college. Since then, he has lived with his parents, and they maintain a close relationship. Mr. D has worked on and off in recent years and remains in contact with a few childhood friends. Although he has no prominent cognitive deficits, and his negative symptoms are mild to moderate in severity, his persistent delusion that he invented the Boeing 747, at times resulting in attempts to gain compensation he believes is his due, interferes with his social and vocational functioning. Mr. D expresses mild dissatisfaction at not having more recreational pursuits, although he enjoys watching TV and going to an occasional ball game with his father or friends.

Over the course of a year, participating in behavioral family therapy and monthly, multiple-family support groups, Mr. D succeeds in achieving two goals: acquiring a job in his area of interest and participating in a greater variety of leisure activities.

Mrs. E is a 27-year-old woman diagnosed with chronic undifferentiated schizophrenia. She lives with her husband, who has alcoholism, and their two children, ages 1 and 4. Mrs. E experiences substantial role strain in attempting to fulfill her responsibilities as a mother. She is easily distracted, which interferes with running a household. Of greater concern, Mrs. E's apathy and anhedonia result in neglect of her children, and child welfare advocates have been called on repeated occasions. Her relationship with her husband is tense as a result of both his intermittent work history complicated by alcohol abuse and her failure to show affection for her family. Mr. and Mrs. E have a circle of friends, including both old high school pals and Mr. E's current drinking buddies. Despite her negative symptoms, Mrs. E expresses a desire to be a better mother and to improve her husband's capacity to work by decreasing his drinking.

Over 2 years of treatment consisting of couples counseling, an alcoholism treatment program and Alcoholics Anonymous (AA) for Mr. E, and both social skills and parenting skills training for Mrs. E, the outlook for the E family changes for the better. Mrs. E's ability to care for her children improves, as does her relationship with her husband. After several unsuccessful attempts to cut down on his alcohol use, Mr. E is now abstinent and has remained so for the past 8 months, and he attends AA meetings regularly. He has worked at the same job for the past 6 months and recently got a raise. Mrs. E still struggles with her apathy but is more successful in achieving personal goals and feels that she has made significant progress.

These vignettes illustrate the complexities of assessing both social functioning and the multiple factors that may impinge on it in the lives of persons with schizophrenia. By definition, social impairments characterize schizophrenia, given that current diagnostic criteria require a disturbance in one or more major areas of functioning, such as work, interpersonal relations, or self-care (American Psychiatric Association 1994). Social functioning has been assessed at many levels, but it is most frequently measured in terms of social roles and social skills. As the vignettes illustrate, both positive and negative symptoms may interfere with optimal fulfillment of social roles such as those of worker or parent. These symptoms—as well as schizophrenia-related neurocognitive deficits and developmental disturbances—can impair social skills and thereby hinder the establishment and fulfillment of social roles.

As this chapter examines social functioning among persons with schizophrenia and related therapeutic interventions, we begin with a brief sketch of social development in schizophrenia and explore how symptom severity, age at onset, and positive and negative symptoms are related to social functioning. We then consider how specific neurocognitive deficits can affect capacities for social functioning and summarize differences in social outcomes across demographic groups. We review interventions designed to overcome social deficits, with an emphasis on social skills training. Finally, we conclude with recommendations for the assessment of improvements in social functioning.

Social Functioning Over the Course of Schizophrenic Illness

Because recruitment for most schizophrenia studies occurs subsequent to first hospitalization, most studies of premorbid social functioning are retrospective. Even prospective studies of high-risk populations cannot always track subtle premorbid changes; nevertheless, there is strong evidence that behavioral, social, and role functioning deficits long precede illness onset. Retrospective parental reports suggest that in childhood, preschizophrenia patients show greater behavioral disruption—including attention and thought problems, social withdrawal, anxious-depressed behavior, and aggression—than do their healthy siblings (Neumann et al. 1995). Retrospective maternal reports describe the social adjustment of schizophrenic patients as deteriorating from childhood through adolescence while that of their siblings improves (McCreadie et al. 1994). Such longitudinal declines in social functioning, assessed retrospectively, are associated more strongly with more pronounced negative symptoms after illness onset (Kelley et al. 1992). One year to 3 years before first onset of psychotic symptoms and 2–4 years before initial hospitalization, social and role function deficits are already evident in more than half of schizophrenic patients (Maurer et al. 1996). By the time of first hospitalization, schizophrenic patients' occupational deficits are more severe than those of affective disorder patients and, unlike the deficits of the latter, occur independently of social stigma, a finding more consistent with biological than with social processes (Beiser et al. 1994). Social adjustment, as measured by the Disability Assessment Schedule (Jablensky et al. 1980), appears to stabilize within 2 years of diagnosis (Mason et al. 1996). Nevertheless, there is considerable heterogeneity in the course of schizophrenia, and social functioning often fails to return to its highest premorbid levels.

Once established in premorbid and prodromal phases of the illness, individuals' relative levels of social functioning remain fairly stable, although acute phases obviously involve acute deterioration in social functioning. Premorbid social adjustment consistently predicts both social and general functioning over the life course (Bailer et al. 1996; Harding et al. 1987a, 1987b; Harrow et al. 1986; Jonsson and Nyman 1991; Rund and Torgalsboen 1990). Number of social relationships prior to first hospitalization consistently predicts both quantity and quality of relationships for several years afterward (Carpenter and Strauss 1991; Strauss and Carpenter 1972, 1974, 1977).

Social Functioning and Expression of Schizophrenic Illness

Illness Severity

Social functioning, as measured by variables such as occupational functioning and community tenure without rehospitalization, has been found to be inversely associated with nearly all indices of illness severity among schizophrenic patients. In addition, it has been linked with poorer prognoses and higher risks for symptom relapse (Johnstone et al. 1990; Perlick et al. 1992; Sullivan et al. 1990) and with more numerous, severe, or persistent symptoms, particularly negative symptoms (Bailer et al. 1996; Breier et al. 1991; Fennig et al. 1995; Keefe et al. 1987; Maurer et al. 1996; Salokangas et al. 1989). Poorer social functioning has also been associated with greater neurocognitive impairment (Dickerson et al. 1996; Green 1996; Ikebuchi et al. 1996), greater chronicity of illness (Jonsson and Nyman 1991), and longer hospitalizations (Bland et al. 1976; Strauss and Carpenter 1974, 1977). Patients with the most pronounced social deficits are more likely to have had premorbid schizophrenia-spectrum personality disturbances (Jonsson and Nyman 1991; McCreadie et al. 1994), an earlier age at illness onset (Harding et al. 1987a, 1987b; Jonsson and Nyman 1991; Rund and Torgelsboen 1990; Schmidt et al. 1995), a more insidious onset (Bailer et al. 1996; Jonsson and Nyman 1991), and a stronger family history of schizophrenia (Keefe et al. 1987; Verdoux et al. 1996). Patients with better social functioning, by contrast, are more likely to have had a voluntary first hospitalization (Rund 1990) and to be of higher socioeconomic status (Gift et al. 1986; Jonsson and Nyman 1991). They are also more likely both to have ever married (McGlashan and Heinssen 1988) and to have been employed in the year prior to first hospitalization (Jonsson and Nyman 1991).

Although the severity of both positive and negative symptoms predicts social functioning, symptom severity may not be the most important practical predictive factor. For example, compared with symptom severity, daily living skills (e.g., hygiene) better predict patients' long-term global outcomes (Jonsson and Nyman 1991) and are more strongly associated with their postdischarge social activity (Tessler and Manderscheid 1982). It therefore appears that, regardless of illness severity, improved community and daily living skills may enhance overall social functioning.

Age at Onset

Younger age at onset of schizophrenia has been associated with more severe symptoms (Maurer et al. 1996; Yang et al. 1995) and poorer social functioning (Maurer et al. 1996), although one study found an unexpected negative association between age at onset and both nonverbal social skills (facial expression, emotional expression, and voice tone) and overall social skills (Ikebuchi et al. 1996). In this sample, however, negative symptoms were also unusually distributed. Nine of 20 patients had teenage onset, and 6 of these 9 showed higher-than-average social skills. All but 1 of these 6 had less-severe negative symptoms than the sample average (Ikebuchi et al. 1996).

Early age at onset not only is an index of illness severity but also contributes directly to social deficits in schizophrenia. Because schizophrenia onset often occurs before either brain maturation or social and cognitive development is complete, it interferes with evolution of social skills appropriate to adult roles (Hafner and Nowotny 1995). As a result of this early onset (earlier than in most other adult psychiatric disorders), schizophrenia has been consistently associated with greater unemployment, less education, and lower lifetime rates of marriage (Keith et al. 1991; Odegaard 1946, 1956, 1960). Interpersonal contact that typically occurs in vocational, educational, and social contexts is thereby diminished and can be further reduced by long hospitalizations (Holmes-Eber and Riger 1990; Lipton et al. 1981). When schizophrenic patients return to the community, social stigma may both weaken their existing social bonds and reduce their likelihood of forming new relationships. Ongoing symptoms such as avolition and anhedonia may further impede initiatives required to establish and fulfill roles of worker and marital partner, as in the case of Mrs. E, described at the beginning of this chapter.

Social Functioning and Symptom Type

Positive Symptoms

At the simplest level, positive symptoms of schizophrenia may interfere with a person's ability to receive information from the external environment, to process it effectively, and to respond appropriately. Positive symptoms have been associated with poor performance on digit-span tasks, which require auditory attention, memory, and sequencing (Berman et al. 1997). Auditory hallucinations affect auditory attention in particular, and thus may disrupt related social functions, such as following the course of a conversation.

Severity of positive symptoms has been associated with poorer social functioning (Keefe et al. 1987; Robins and Guze 1970). Positive symptoms sometimes have been associated with social phobia and agoraphobia (Penn et al. 1994), dysphoria (Lysaker et al. 1995a; Mueser et al. 1991c), and psychosocial stressors (Peralta et al. 1995). Patients with positive symptoms such as delusions and hallucinations tend to have lower global assessment of functioning scores and more hospitalizations (Peralta et al. 1995). In the case example of Mr. D (presented at the beginning of this chapter), the patient's tendency to discuss his delusional belief that he had invented the Boeing 747 interfered with both work and family relationships. Although his firm conviction in this belief did not change, Mr. D learned to improve his social relationships by refraining from introducing it into conversation.

However, positive symptoms seem to interfere with social functioning less than negative symptoms do (Pogue-Geile and Harrow 1984). In fact, one study that controlled for the effects of negative symptoms eliminated all significant effects of positive symptoms on social functioning, although both negative and positive symptoms continued to make independent contributions to global social functioning (Breier et al. 1991). Compared with schizophrenic patients with prominent negative symptoms, those with positive symptoms show higher levels of residential independence and are more likely to report a range of leisure activities (C. A. Harvey et al. 1996). However, when positive symptoms co-occur with negative symptoms, they usually reflect greater illness severity than do negative symptoms occurring alone. For example, visual hallucinations are related to poorer mental status and occupational outcome (Coryell and Tsuang 1986) and, unlike other forms of hallucinations, are significantly associated with global severity of illness (Mueser et al. 1990a). Patients with either mixed positive and negative symptoms or only negative symptoms function more poorly before hospitalization and stay longer in the hospital than do patients with only positive symptoms (Pogue-Geile and Harrow 1984). However, patients with only negative symptoms are less likely to complete high school than those with either mixed symptoms or only positive symptoms (Pogue-Geile and Harrow 1984). Negative symptoms, whether alone or in combination with positive symptoms, are associated with poorer premorbid social and educational functioning and may therefore serve as a more reliable index of illness severity than positive symptoms.

Negative Symptoms

Although negative symptoms have been consistently associated with psychopathological severity and poorer social functioning (Bailer et al. 1996; Breier et al. 1991; Keefe et al. 1987; Maurer et al. 1996; Robins and Guze 1970; Salokangas et al. 1989), these observed relationships may be inflated by conceptual overlap. Studies controlling for such overlap, however, still show a strong association between social deficits and those negative symptoms not typically included in measures of social functioning, such as affective blunting and alogia (Maurer et al. 1996).

One advantage of considering negative symptoms in relationship to social functioning is that these symptoms are fairly specific to schizophrenia (Cuesta and Peralta 1995). Negative symptoms occur only infrequently in other psychiatric disorders (Pogue-Geile and Harrow 1984), and when they occur outside of schizophrenia (e.g., in affective psychosis), they have little prognostic value (Husted et al. 1995). They do not appear to endure except in schizophrenia (Husted et al. 1995), and their presence during nonacute phases adds to their potential prognostic importance (Pogue-Geile and Harrow 1984). Negative symptoms show greater stability than positive symptoms, which suggests that they represent a core feature of schizophrenia (Eaton et al. 1995; McGlashan and Fenton 1992; Mueser et al. 1991c).

Because negative symptoms are associated with most measures of illness severity (e.g., earlier age at onset, poorer neuroleptic response, increased likelihood of premorbid schizoid or schizotypal personality disorder [Chaves et al. 1993; Peralta et al. 1995]), they are also related to a developmental course of social difficulties. Stable (versus unstable) negative symptoms in adulthood are associated with poorer premorbid social relationships (Fennig et al. 1995) as well as with poorer pre-onset adjustment and worse post-onset outcomes (Bailer et al. 1996; Gupta et al. 1995; Larsen et al.1996; Mueser et al. 1990c; Pogue-Geile 1989; Vazquez-Barquero et al. 1996). The presence of negative symptoms at illness onset predicts social disability at 3 years after first hospitalization (Maurer et al. 1996). Negative symptoms are also related to reduced social competence (Bellack et al. 1990b; Jackson et al. 1989; Lysaker and Bell 1995; Mueser et al. 1990a; Solinski et al. 1992) and to impairments in both vocational and avocational pursuits and in social problem solving (Bellack et al. 1994; Corrigan et al. 1994; Davidson and McGlashan 1997; C. A. Harvey et al. 1996; Hoffman and Kupper 1997).

The "disorder of relating" construct, which includes the negative symptoms of avoidance and withdrawal, shows strong negative associations with social functioning, surpassing social skills as a predictor of work performance in a role-play test (Hoffman and Kupper 1997). Specific "disorder of relating" symptoms also show strong individual associations with social and occupational function. Psychomotor retardation (C. A. Harvey et al. 1996), social withdrawal (Coryell and Tsuang 1986), and poverty of speech (Pogue-Geile and Harrow 1984), for example, are all associated with poorer occupational outcome. Psychomotor poverty is also associated with fewer leisure activities (C. A. Harvey et al. 1996). Anergia has been associated with nonverbal-paralinguistic skill and with overall social skill, but not with verbal content (Mueser et al. 1996), which suggests that this symptom interferes more with nonverbal social abilities than with verbal ones. Although the presence of negative symptoms consistently predicts poorer social function, not all poorly functioning schizophrenic patients present with negative symptoms (Pogue-Geile and Harrow 1984).

Negative symptoms are not a unitary construct. For example, deficits in affective response, long considered pathognomonic of schizophrenia (Bleuler 1911/1950; Kraepelin 1919/1971), may actually represent two different dimensions, one of experience and another of expression. The distinction between these dimensions is supported by factor analyses in which social amotivation and diminished expression emerged as indices of separate, distinct factors (Sayers et al. 1996) and by numerous studies showing incongruity between schizophrenic patients' affective experience and their affective expression (Berenbaum and Oltmanns 1992; Berenbaum et al. 1987; Kring and Neale 1996). Schizophrenic patients, particularly those with blunted affect, show less facial expression than do nonschizophrenic patients but report experiencing equally intense emotion (Berenbaum and Oltmanns 1992; Berenbaum et al. 1987). In fact, while viewing films designed to elicit a wide range of emotion, schizophrenic patients in one study showed greater skin conductance reactivity than did nonschizophrenic control subjects (Kring and Neale 1996), suggesting that schizophrenic patients either experience certain affects more intensely or show more generalized autonomic hyperresponsivity than controls (Dawson and Nuechterlein 1984). This disjunction of experienced and expressed affect may impair social relationships insofar as persons who interact with schizophrenic patients are likely to underestimate these patients' emotional experiences, particularly in the presence of severe blunted affect (Blanchard and Panzarella 1998).

Diminished affective expression in speech often accompanies blunted facial affect (Andreasen et al. 1981). Certain speech anomalies are specific to schizophrenia, and although no single pattern characterizes all schizophrenic patients, well over half speak with either constricted timbre (volume), narrowed range of pitch, or both (Stein 1993). In normal speech, minimal volume inflection often indicates social unavailablility, and the absence of pitch inflection conveys either disinterest or lack of emotion (Stein 1993). The muting and restriction of melodic range of schizophrenic speech may interfere with social interactions, since vocal volume and tone can fail to convey the actual level of experienced emotion. Parallel to findings in studies of facial affective expression, patients with restrictions of timbre and pitch experience more intense affect than their vocal expression would suggest (Stein 1993).

Anhedonia, long recognized to be a factor in the development of schizophrenia (Meehl 1962), appears to mediate the relationship between risk for schizophrenia and later social dysfunction (Freedman et al. 1998). Patients either with or without affective expression deficits may experience anhedonia. Anhedonia interferes primarily with affectively positive interpersonal interactions. In a study in which schizophrenia patients were asked to view films with both positive and negative content, patients scoring high on physical anhedonia reported less positive mood than did those scoring lower on this factor (Blanchard et al. 1994). Anhedonia has also been associated with poorer social skills (Beckfield 1985; Haberman et al. 1979; Numbers and Chapman 1982), but only in affiliative interactions, not in conflictual ones (Blanchard et al. 1994). It should also be noted that anhedonia in schizophrenia patients has been linked with neuroleptic use (Harrow et al. 1994); for this reason, the effects of pharmacological treatments should be considered when evaluating this symptom.

Schizophrenia Symptoms, Neurocognitive Impairments, and Social Functioning

Given that social cognition is built upon nonsocial information-processing abilities such as attention, memory, and executive functions (Penn et al. 1997), it is not surprising that neurocognitive factors play an important role in social competence (Liberman et al. 1986; McFall 1982; Spaulding et al. 1986). Penn and colleagues (1997) estimated from a meta-analysis of previous studies that nonsocial information processing accounts for nearly 25% of the variance in social competence in schizophrenia, although the relationship between nonsocial cognition and social functioning appears to be stronger among female than male patients (Mueser et al. 1995; Penn et al. 1996).

Neurocognitive deficits are generally established at schizophrenia onset and remain stable, with neither marked deterioration nor improvement over time (Davidson and McGlashan 1997; Hyde et al. 1994; Roy and DeVriendt 1994). They often appear long before the onset of illness, and longitudinal relationships between neurocognitive and social deficits are bidirectional. The presence of premorbid childhood and adolescent neurological symptoms is associated with poorer adulthood social functioning in schizophrenic patients (Jonsson and Nyman 1991), and premorbid childhood social deficits predict adulthood neurocognitive symptoms (Baum and Walker 1995).

Neurocognitive impairments often accompany negative symptoms (Davidson and McGlashan 1997; Roy and DeVriendt 1994) and may mediate some of the associations observed between negative symptoms and social function. In fact, negative symptoms are more strongly related to certain neurocognitive functions, such as difficulty in abstract thinking, than to certain social ones, such as social withdrawal (McCreadie et al. 1994), and neurocognitive functioning is more consistently related to social functioning than is symptomatology (Green 1996). Neurocognitive processes appear not only to mediate the effects of symptoms on social functioning but also to moderate them in a compensatory way. For example, symptomatic schizophrenic patients may process social information differently than do both healthy and psychiatric control subjects. In a hinting task, schizophrenic patients were less able than controls to infer true intentions from indirect speech, suggesting that perspective-taking may be particularly difficult for them when others' communications are indirect (Corcoran et al. 1995). However, hinting task performance and IQ were highly correlated among schizophrenic patients but not among controls, suggesting that schizophrenic patients rely more than controls do on generalized intellectual abilities to infer the mental states of others (Corcoran et al. 1995).

Patients with the most severe cognitive impairments show the most persistent deficits in social skills (Lysaker et al. 1995b). This finding reflects more than better functioning with stronger general intelligence; specific neurocognitive deficits are differentially associated with specific dimensions of social cognition and functioning, although this sometimes reflects a differential sensitivity of specific psychometric instruments (Penn et al. 1995). For example, whereas social functioning was not significantly related to neuropsychological measures when measured with rating scales (Brekke et al. 1997), it showed significant associations when measured with role-play data (Penn et al. 1995). Nevertheless, two specific measures of neurocognitive function—secondary verbal memory and card-sorting tasks—have demonstrated consistent relationships with social and occupational functioning across numerous studies (Green 1996).

General Verbal and Nonverbal Abilities

One way to categorize the influence of neurocognitive deficits on social functioning is in terms of verbal and nonverbal abilities, such as those measured by standard IQ tests. Verbal learning is associated with general social skills (Kern et al. 1992) and with more specific skills in emotion recognition (Bryson et al. 1997). The verbal portion of the Wechsler Memory Scale–Revised (Wechsler 1987) predicts social role-play performance (Mueser et al. 1991a), and verbal memory is associated with functional outcomes in schizophrenia (Green 1996). Although a wealth of literature examines schizophrenia-related deficits in receptive and expressive language, little of it focuses specifically on social outcomes. Nonetheless, it is reasonable to hypothesize that such communication deficits also hinder social interaction.

Nonverbal abilities are also associated with social functioning among schizophrenic patients. Performance IQ correlates significantly with the receiving and processing of social information and with global social skills (Ikebuchi et al. 1996). McEvoy et al. (1996) found that a variety of parietal functions, as measured by tasks such as the Judgment of Line Orientation test (Benton et al. 1983), the Block Design subtest of the Wechsler Adult Intelligence Scale–Revised (WAIS-R; Wechsler 1981), the Rey-Osterrieth Complex Figure Test (Osterrieth 1944; Rey 1942), the Finger Localization test (Benton et al. 1983), and a general Parietal Factor score, were associated with social knowledge.

Visual memory deficits, evidenced in poorer-than-average performance in picture completion tasks (Crookes 1984), are also related to social deficits, and better complex visuomotor processing is associated with improved work functioning and independent living skills (Brekke et al. 1997). Schizophrenic patients show particular deficits in tasks of facial recognition, and these difficulties may account for their difficulties in identifying emotions from others' facial expressions (Kerr and Neale 1993; Mueser et al. 1996). Performance on face perception tests is related to social competence, including social adjustment on the ward and social skill, as well as to illness severity, age at first hospitalization, duration of hospitalization, and presence of anergia (Mueser et al. 1996).

Reaction Time and Arousal

One of the most consistent findings in the neurocognitive literature is of slower reaction times among schizophrenic patients. Patients with shorter reaction times show better responses to psychiatric rehabilitation (Wykes et al. 1990), better paralinguistic skills in role plays, and better social problem-solving skills (Penn et al. 1995). At the most basic level, the psychophysiological arousal and responses measured in reaction-time experiments are fundamental to attention, which, in turn, is fundamental to many higher-order social functions.

Higher levels of resting arousal and better orienting responses (as measured by skin conductance), for example, are associated with better scores on social outcome and role function scales (Brekke et al. 1997).

Measures of brain-wave activity related to attentional processes are also associated with social functioning outcomes: N1 wave amplitudes, which are related to sensory function and selective attention, show a significant association with nonverbal social skills, as does N1 latency with global social skills (Ikebuchi et al. 1996). By contrast, more traditional neuropsychological measures (e.g., Stroop, digit symbol, block design, verbal fluency) bear no relationship to social outcome or role function, but rather are associated with employment or independent living, which, in turn, show no relationship to arousal and orienting responses (Brekke et al. 1997). This evidence suggests that whereas schizophrenic patients' impairments in social interaction skills are proportional to their deficits in fundamental orienting processes, their success in employment and independent living is more strongly reliant on mastery of instrumental tasks for which other neurocognitive skills are necessary (Brekke et al. 1997).

Early Information Processing

Early information processing is processing that occurs within the first few seconds of a stimulus presentation; it involves attention, memory, and the ability to distinguish between relevant and irrelevant stimuli. This ability is generally assessed with tasks that require immediate responses to a series of stimuli, such as the span of apprehension task, in which a series of digits is presented and a response is required when a target digit appears (Penn et al. 1995). Impairments in early information processing probably result from an inability to represent stimuli internally for current and future use (Cohen and Servan-Schreiber 1993), from working-memory deficits (Goldman-Rakic 1992), and from deficits in vigilance (Elkins et al. 1992). Deficits in early information processing predict social dysfunction in individuals at risk for schizophrenia (Cornblatt et al. 1992; Cornblatt and Kelip 1994; Erlenmeyer-Kimling et al. 1993) and reduced global social competence in schizophrenic patients (Penn et al. 1995). Specific social skills that require early information processing include following a conversational topic, remembering important interpersonal information, and attending to relevant social cues.

Contextual Processing

Early information processing includes some aspects of contextual processing. An inability to discriminate between relevant and irrelevant information may impair social functioning because social behavior involves both perception of relevant social cues and initiation of appropriate responses. Experimental evidence shows that schizophrenic patients fail to evaluate information accurately on a consistent basis and use less effective strategies for screening out irrelevant information (Niwa et al. 1992). Their responses to stimuli are often delayed, suggesting difficulties in both stimulus evaluation and response organization, as well as some disjunction between the stimulus evaluation process and the response organization process (Niwa et al. 1992). Impairments in differentiating between target and irrelevant stimuli are observed in both auditory and visual tasks and therefore are not modality specific (Harris et al. 1985). In a study of schizophrenic patients' performance on a free-association task of word pairs, number and severity of psychiatric symptoms correlated significantly with number of contextually inappropriate responses (Allen 1990). Although these contextual errors showed no association with premorbid IQ, marital status, education, or duration of personal relationships, they were associated with poorer employment history.

Memory

Schizophrenia appears to interfere with active, effortful processing of information (Nuechterlein and Dawson 1984), and in the passive processing of information, the failure to establish and maintain set interferes with both memory and attention (Carter and Flesher 1995; Hogarty and Flesher 1992). Memory impairment in schizophrenia is significantly associated with negative symptoms but not with age, IQ, positive symptoms, or general psychopathology (Stirling et al. 1997). Although memory deficits characteristic of schizophrenia were not widely observed in his sample, Tsuang (1982) found that patients who experienced such deficits also had poorer marital and occupational outcomes. More severe memory impairments, like more severe negative symptoms, may simply reflect general severity of illness, which would include severe social deficits. However, there is also evidence that specific memory deficits contribute to specific difficulties in social functioning. Social inference, for example, requires memory of past contexts in order to interpret new situations, and therefore relies specifically on episodic memory.

Attentional Processes

A large literature attests to the presence of attentional deficits among patients with schizophrenia and their first-degree relatives, particularly in the abilities to maintain attention, to follow and remember sequences, and to ignore irrelevant input (Cornblatt et al. 1997; Nuechterlein and Dawson 1984; Mirsky and Duncan 1986; Mirsky et al. 1992; Morice and Delahunty 1996; Weintraub 1987). One categorization of attentional processes separates them into four areas: encoding, focus and execution, sustained attention, and cognitive flexibility (i.e., the ability to shift attention) (Mirsky et al. 1995).

Focus and Execution

The ability to focus on stimuli and respond appropriately is assessed with tasks such as Digit-Symbol Substitution from the WAIS-R, the Stroop Word-Color Interference Test (Stroop 1935), the Talland Letter Cancellation Test (Lezak 1976), and the Trail Making Test (Reitan 1985). Both schizophrenic patients and their relatives with psychiatric diagnoses perform more poorly than control participants from the community on these tasks (Mirsky et al. 1995). Digit-symbol tasks, which require the substitution of abstract symbols for numbers, are associated with emotion recognition (Bryson et al. 1997). Poor differentiation between colors and words in the Stroop task has been associated with communication deviance (i.e., oddly worded, unclear, and fragmented speech) (Velligan et al. 1997), selective-attention deficits, and poor reality monitoring (Brebion et al. 1996).

Sustained Attention

The continuous performance task (CPT), in which patients are asked to identify a target stimulus from a series of presented stimuli, measures sustained attention (Mirsky et al. 1995) and is associated with motor speed and variability of response latencies (van den Bosch et al. 1996). In schizophrenic patients, poorer CPT performance is also associated with negative symptoms and formal thought disorder (Nuechterlein et al. 1986). Also known as vigilance or directed attention, sustained attention is consistently associated with social problem-solving skills and with social skills acquisition among schizophrenic patients (Bowen et al. 1994; Corrigan et al. 1994; Kern et al. 1992; Penn et al. 1993, 1995), as well as with better medication management (Corrigan et al. 1994). Schizophrenic patients who can distinguish signal from background on the CPT also show better affect recognition, because they are more able to discriminate facial expression and tone of voice from spoken words (Bryson et al. 1997). Presumably, signal detection—specifically, discrimination of nonverbal and paralinguistic cues—underlies more complex social cognition. Although, historically, affective and social deficits in schizophrenia have been conceptualized as separate domains, the two are inextricably linked (Dworkin 1992), as both require the ability to assess voice and tone accurately during spoken communication (paralinguistic features), to perceive nonverbal cues correctly, and to discriminate emotions based on the verbal content of speech. Affect recognition is also associated with scores on the Wisconsin Card Sorting Test (WCST; Heaton 1981), the Wechsler Memory Scale figural memory subscale, and recognition of true positives on the Hopkins Verbal Learning Test (Brandt 1991) (Bryson et al. 1997). These data suggest that affect recognition is related not only to sustained attention but also to cognitive flexibility, visual memory, and contextual processing.

Cognitive Flexibility

Cognitive flexibility is most often measured by performance on the WCST. Compared with nonpsychiatric control subjects, schizophrenic patients show significantly more perseverative errors on the WCST, indicating impairments in cognitive flexibility and planning (Morice 1990; Morice and Delahunty 1996). These impairments, although not related to WAIS-R IQ data (Morice and Delahunty 1996) or social problem solving (Green 1996), are associated with poorer community functioning (Green 1996).

Executive Function

Executive function deficits are associated with poorer social adjustment (Jaeger and Douglas 1992). On the Tower of London task (Shallice 1982), schizophrenic patients require more moves to complete an arrangement, and solve significantly fewer rearrangements in the predetermined number of moves, than do nonpsychiatric control subjects (Morris et al. 1995). Inaccurate planning, which does not vary by symptomatology, appears to be the cause of this poorer performance (Morris et al. 1995). Deficits in executive function seem to interfere with the ability to plan effectively for social behavior, thus compromising social functioning. Furthermore, schizophrenic patients show a disproportionate decline in performance as tasks become longer and more complex (Morice and Delahunty 1996), which suggests that extended and multifaceted interpersonal interactions may be particularly taxing for them.

Abstraction and Conceptual Organization

Persons with schizophrenia also have specific difficulties with abstract features of social situations, such as understanding the goals of specific behaviors, particularly when presented with an unfamiliar situation (Corrigan and Green 1993; Corrigan et al. 1996). Such difficulties in abstraction may lead to misreading of social contexts and the motivations of others. Conceptual disorganization, which can result from more general problems with abstraction, can impair the ability to learn and is related to work performance in schizophrenic patients (Hoffman and Kupper 1997).

Differences in Social Functioning Across Demographic and Subdiagnostic Groups

Age at Onset

In studies conducted in the 1970s, younger schizophrenic patients showed better social adjustment than older patients (Bland et al. 1976, 1978). This finding seems counterintuitive, given that earlier age at onset is generally more prevalent among males and is associated with more severe schizophrenia. Given that social skills are higher among female patients, one might expect younger groups to contain more severe, chronic cases and a higher proportion of males, both of which would be associated with poorer social functioning. The finding of better social adjustment among younger patients may therefore reflect biological and social processes by which social deficits increase over time, although such declines in function have not been the norm. It is more likely that this finding represents a cohort effect. In recent years, younger patients have generally received more effective medication earlier in treatment, which can arrest deteriorative processes associated with untreated or poorly treated schizophrenia. In more recent studies, older schizophrenic patients show better social skills than in older studies (Mueser et al. 1990c), a finding consistent with a longitudinal trend for earlier, more effective treatment of schizophrenia.

Gender

Schizophrenic patients' sex differences in social functioning may be associated with sex differences in neuropsychological functioning. When compared, respectively, with controls of their own sex, male schizophrenic patients showed impairments across all neuropsychological functions, whereas female patients showed deficits only in the areas of attention, executive functions, visual memory, and motor functions (Goldstein et al. 1998). Schizophrenic patients differ by sex in the areas of social competence (Mueser et al. 1990b; Perry et al. 1995), social adjustment (Smith et al. 1997), and social functioning (Fennig et al. 1995), with women showing fewer impairments in these areas than men. In the area of social skills, however, there is an interaction between gender and participation in social skills training, with increasing levels of participation in skills training leading to much greater improvement in males than in females (Smith et al. 1997). Nevertheless, female patients receiving social skills training show lower negative symptom totals at discharge—specifically, in the symptoms of alogia, avolition, and flat affect (Smith et al. 1997). These benefits are similar to those experienced by Mrs. E (described at the beginning of this chapter), whose participation in social skills training resulted in improved relationships with her husband and children and a concomitant reduction in apathy and social anhedonia.

This sex difference in social skills training outcomes must be interpreted in light of two possible confounds, however. First, because schizophrenia onset occurs earlier in males than it does in females, the development of adult social skills may be more disrupted for men than for women. Therefore, men's baseline social functioning may be more impaired than women's, and this factor may account, in part, for male patients' disproportionate improvement with social skills training. Second, gender differences in social functioning are not specific to schizophrenia: such differences have also been found in the general population. For example, there is evidence of an imprinted, X-linked genetic locus related to social cognition and behavior, wherein women receive one active and one inactive allele, and men, only one, inactive allele. The effect of this differential distribution is to render women more naturally adept in certain areas of social functioning (Skuse et al. 1997; McGuffin and Scourfield 1997).

Although there is evidence for gender differences in social functioning among schizophrenic patients, the relative influence of sex on outcome may vary. For example, in a recent international study, the differential effects of gender on outcome were not as great as the effects of research center (or nation/society), marital status, and premorbid personality traits (Jablensky and Cole 1997). The effects on outcome of family history of psychiatric disorder appeared to be comparable to those of gender but remained nonsignificant because of greater variability (Jablensky and Cole 1997).

Marital Status

Epidemiological studies have consistently found higher rates of never marrying among schizophrenic patients than among any other Axis I diagnostic group (Odegaard 1946) except that of substance abuse (Robins et al. 1991), which contains an overrepresentation of young adults who have not passed the age of greatest "risk" for marriage. This lower rate of marriage among schizophrenic patients has often been attributed to the fact that the onset age of schizophrenia precedes the usual ages of marriage in the general population. Indeed, compared with never-married patients, ever-married patients are generally older at illness onset and less severely ill. Although marital status may be a social outcome of age at onset and illness severity, it may also contribute to other social outcomes, given that marriage may provide both a source of social support and access to a wider social network.

Age at Onset, Gender, and Marital Status

Evidence suggests that whereas age at onset of schizophrenia is unrelated to marriage in men, women with a late onset of schizophrenia are significantly more likely to marry than their early-onset counterparts (Lewine et al. 1997). This finding probably reflects more than a simple sex difference in the relationship between age at onset and marriage. It should be interpreted with caution in light of the gender differences in complexity of developmental processes (which may interfere with marriage prior to illness onset), expectations for courtship, and ages of marriage in the general population.

In an Indian sample of married schizophrenic patients living with their spouses, women showed greater disability than men, a difference attributed to conditions of Indian society (Shankar et al. 1995) but also attributable to age-at-onset differences. Women generally experience illness onset at a later age than do men and are more likely to marry, regardless of their ultimate level of impairment. Married women with schizophrenia thus may not differ significantly from nonmarried women with schizophrenia in terms of illness severity. Male schizophrenia patients who are married, however, may be less impaired than those who are nonmarried, given that their symptoms neither occurred early enough in life nor were severe enough to interfere with the formation of a marital relationship. Data from the World Health Organization suggest that determinants of marriage among schizophrenic patients differ by gender across multiple societies, with age at onset and good premorbid adjustment best predicting marriage for men, and age at onset and supportive social environment best predicting it for women (Jablensky and Cole 1997). Indeed, both raw and adjusted differences in mean age at onset between nonmarried and married individuals were larger for men than for women across most cultures, as well as in the total sample (Jablensky and Cole 1997).

Therapeutic Interventions

Just as social functioning in schizophrenia may be addressed at multiple levels of individual and collective behaviors, interventions to improve social functioning have been attempted at many levels. Some interventions involve reme-diation of very specific neurocognitive deficits, such as attention problems. Others focus on social skills training to improve interpersonal functioning. Family therapy aims at reducing tension in the family environment and empowering family members to cope with the illness. Social network inter-ventions generally seek to broaden and increase the efficacy of the patient's social network, and supported employment programs try to help patients acquire competitive jobs and function better in work settings, thereby promoting their integration into the larger community.

Cognitive Remediation Interventions

Interventions aimed at specific neurocognitive deficits, whether used alone or in combination with other interventions, have been demonstrated to improve patients' social performance in controlled studies. Attention-focused social training has enhanced conversation skills (Massell et al. 1991), and vigilance and memory training have improved perception of social cues (Corrigan et al. 1995). Other therapies designed to enhance cognitive functioning, such as scaffolding instruction designed to boost performance on the WCST (Young and Freyslinger 1995), may also improve both cognitive flexibility and social interactions that require maintaining and shifting set, such as following a conversation. However, the more generalized effects of cognitive remediation on social functioning have not been established.

Family Interventions

Family interventions for schizophrenia have focused on reducing tension in the family, educating family members about schizophrenia, and empowering the family to cope better with the effects of the illness. Family intervention programs following this model and providing at least 9 months of treatment have significantly reduced rates either of relapse or of rehospitalization over 18–24 months (Baucom et al. 1998). Controlled studies comparing multiple-family versus single-family treatments have reported similar reductions in relapse and rehospitalization (Baucom et al. 1998).

Social Skills Interventions

The concept of social skills has evolved in recent years to identify the deter-minants of adequate social role functioning. Social skills can be defined as those specific abilities that enable individuals to achieve instrumental (e.g., purchasing an item at a store) and affiliative (e.g., making friends) goals in an interpersonal context (Liberman et al. 1989). Whereas *social skills* refers to the specific abilities necessary to achieve these goals, *social competence* refers to the actual attainment of these goals or the ability to meet societally defined role expectations (Mueser et al. 1990c).

Social skills are divided into three broad types: social perception skills, cognitive skills, and behavioral skills (Wallace et al. 1980). This tripartite conceptualization is based on the assumption that effective social behavior requires individuals to perceive relevant situational parameters (e.g., recognition of the other person's emotion), formulate goals and select strategies for attaining those goals, and enact these strategic plans through appropriate use of paralinguistic, nonverbal, and verbal skills.

The hypothesis that social skills contribute to social functioning has been supported by several studies. Bellack et al. (1990a) showed that role-play assessments of social skill among schizophrenic patients were related to independent measures of social functioning in the community. In a study of inpatients with chronic schizophrenia, Penn and colleagues (1995) reported that social skills, as rated with an unstructured conversation probe, were significantly correlated with independent ratings of ward behavior. Finally, in a study of patients with schizophrenia, Appelo and colleagues (1992) found that specific social behavior, as assessed by simulated social interactions, was significantly correlated with staff's independent global ratings of social competence based on observations of ward behavior.

Research demonstrating that social skills performance tends to be related to other correlates of social functioning provides further evidence for the validity of the social skills construct. Specifically, social skills impairments tend to be more pronounced in individuals with schizophrenia than in individuals with affective disorders or with no psychiatric disorder (Bellack et al. 1990b, 1992; Mueser et al. 1991a, 1995). Social skills deficits are also more prevalent among males (Bellack et al. 1992; Mueser et al. 1990b, 1995), among patients with more prominent negative symptoms (Appelo et al. 1992; Jackson et al. 1989; Lysaker et al. 1995b; Mueser et al. 1991c), and among those with more severe cognitive deficits (Bellack et al. 1994; Mueser et al. 1991b; Penn et al. 1995).

Controlled studies of social skills interventions for patients with schizophrenia have shown that these interventions are more effective than control treatments in reducing symptoms and improving social adjustment, although not in reducing relapse rates (see Penn and Mueser 1996 for a review). In general, social skills training has been more effective when provided over a longer period (at least 1 year), and it is associated with greater improvements in specific social behaviors than in either symptoms or community functioning. There is evidence, however, that social skills training is more effective than milieu therapy in reducing negative symptoms at 6 months (Dobson et al. 1995) and that patients with an earlier age at onset experience greater improvements in social skills than do those with a later illness onset (Marder et al. 1996).

Recommendations for Assessment of Improvements in Social Functioning

As we have reviewed in this chapter, social functioning may be influenced by a variety of illness-related and independent environmental factors. To improve the social adjustment of persons with schizophrenia, valid and reliable measures of social functioning are necessary. In recent years there has been a proliferation of instruments designed to evaluate social functioning in schizophrenia and other severe mental illnesses. A comprehensive review of these instruments is provided by Scott and Lehman (1998).

These instruments vary in format, ranging from interview-based measures and rating scales to self-report instruments and role-play tests of social and problem-solving skill. Interview measures of social functioning, especially when they also tap the perceptions of caregivers such as family members, tend to provide the highest level of specificity in terms of patient social behavior and deficits, and therefore are quite useful in treatment planning and outcome evaluation. The primary limitation of these instruments is that they are time-consuming to administer, usually requiring at least 1 hour of direct interviewing with the client and often more. Examples of interview-based instruments are the Social Adjustment Scale II (Schooler et al. 1978), the Social Dysfunction Index (Munroe-Blum et al. 1996), and the Cardinal Needs Survey (Marshall et al. 1995).

Rating scales are designed to be completed by a provider or family member who is familiar with the patient. Measures vary in length and specificity, ranging from relatively brief assessments requiring global ratings (e.g., the Multnomah Community Ability Scale [Barker et al. 1994a, 1994b]) to more comprehensive scales (e.g., the Social Behavior Schedule [Wykes and Sturt 1986], the Social-Adaptive Functioning Evaluation [P. D. Harvey et al. 1997]). Although less time-consuming than interview-based assessments, rating scales usually provide less specificity as well, and they may be less sensitive to the effects of treatment.

The utility of self-report instruments in persons with schizophrenia remains unclear, at least in part because of the neuropsychological deficits so common in the disorder (Scott and Lehman 1998). Role-play assessments of social and problem-solving skills (see Bellack et al. 1997) provide critical information for the identification and remediation of specific skills deficits, but they do not measure social functioning (i.e., role functioning) per se. Overall, the optimal approach to the measurement of social functioning includes both interview-based and provider-based assessments. To the extent that skills-training approaches are used to improve social functioning, role-play measures are helpful and provide a high level of behavioral specificity; such measures can therefore be employed to evaluate a program's success in improving targeted social skills.

We conclude with specific recommendations for assessing improvements in social functioning over the course of schizophrenia.

1. Identify areas of role functioning in which the patient has failed to live up to others' or his/her own expectations. Impairments in self-care skills and in fulfillment of social roles (e.g., student, parent, worker) are common problem areas. In which areas of role functioning is the patient motivated to improve? Evaluate changes in the quality and enjoyment of interpersonal relationships and leisure and recreational time. Although social roles and leisure activities represent different areas of functioning, they are strongly interrelated, and deficits in one area are often associated with deficits in the other. When evaluating improvements in interpersonal relationships, attend both to patients' perceptions of the quality of these relationships and to their satisfaction with them, as well as to undesired social isolation. To determine whether improvements have occurred in leisure and recreational activities, explore the activities formerly engaged in but subsequently discontinued by the patient, as well as any new areas he or she has identified.

2. Determine whether the supportiveness or affective tone of family members in close contact with the patient has changed. High levels of criticism, emotional overinvolvement (e.g., intrusiveness, lack of objectivity, extreme self-sacrificing behavior), and hostility are especially pernicious, although warmth and appreciation of the patient may mitigate some of the negative effects of these other emotions. Observe behaviors in meetings with individual family members and the family as a whole to evaluate whether improvements have occurred in domains such as supportiveness or negativity.

3. Assess whether the patient's other social networks have expanded or become more supportive. Some patients have small and highly intercon-

nected networks, whereas others have larger, less dense networks. Evaluate changes in both the size of the network and the extent of reciprocity. Patients with high levels of dependency tend to have social networks in which they receive numerous contacts and benefits but provide few benefits to others, creating strained relationships. Increasing the reciprocity of relationships increases satisfaction with social contacts on the part of both patients and others.

4. Assess changes in the severity of negative symptoms, positive symptoms, and cognitive deficits and the contributions of these changes to social functioning. Although symptoms and cognitive deficits are only moderately correlated with social functioning, interventions that target specific coping skills or compensatory strategies can decrease the untoward effects of symptoms and cognitive deficits on social functioning. For example, problems with focused attention can interfere with performance in the workplace. Patients who have been taught to take regular breaks on the job may demonstrate improved work performance. Similarly, patients who learn strategies for managing persistent positive symptoms, such as interacting with others, listening to music on headphones, or humming when auditory hallucinations become severe, may show improvement in their social functioning. To evaluate such changes, clinicians should focus on assessing both the presence of new coping or compensatory skills and their associated impact on social functioning.

5. Evaluate changes in specific social skills deficits. Poor performance in areas such as eye contact, facial expressiveness, vocal tone, and appropriateness of verbal content can contribute to problems in social relationships. To determine whether social skills have improved, assessments should focus on specific skills in specific situations and should take into account the goals of both the patient and significant others, the extent of the patient's cognitive deficits, the mores of the cultural group to which the patient belongs, medication side effects, and the social environment in which the patient resides. When blunted affect is a prominent symptom and nonverbal expressions are thereby muted, clinicians should evaluate whether the patient has learned to express feelings verbally so as to avoid the common social misunderstanding that patients with diminished expressiveness experience few emotions.

Conclusions

Social deficits that accompany schizophrenia are related to severity of illness as well as to specific symptoms and neurocognitive deficits. Interventions that specifically address social skills, as well as those that address underlying neurocognitive and symptom-related impairments and those that address work and community integration, can improve social functioning in ways that enhance quality of life for schizophrenic patients and their families.

References

Allen H: Cognitive processing and its relationship to symptoms and social functioning in schizophrenia. Br J Psychiatry 156:201–203, 1990

American Psychiatric Association: Diagnostic and Statistical Manual of Mental Disorders, 4th Edition. Washington, DC, American Psychiatric Association, 1994

Andreasen NC, Alpert MK, Martz MJ: Acoustic analysis: an objective measure of affective flattening. Arch Gen Psychiatry 38:281–285, 1981

Appelo MT, Woonings FMJ, van Nieuwenhuizen CJ, et al: Specific skills and social competence in schizophrenia. Acta Psychiatr Scand 85:419–422, 1992

Bailer J, Brauer W, Rey ER: Premorbid adjustment as predictor of outcome in schizophrenia: Results of a prospective study. Acta Psychiatr Scand 93:368–377, 1996

Barker S, Barron N, McFarland BH, et al: A Community Ability Scale for chronically mentally ill consumers, part I: reliability and validity. Community Ment Health J 30:363–383, 1994a

Barker S, Barron N, McFarland BH, et al: A Community Ability Scale for chronically mentally ill consumers, part II: applications. Community Ment Health J 30:459–472, 1994b

Baucom DH, Shoham V, Mueser KT, et al: Empirically supported couple and family interventions for marital distress and adult mental health problems. J Consult Clin Psychol 66:53–88, 1998

Baum KM, Walker EF: Childhood behavioral precursors of adult symptom dimensions in schizophrenia. Schizophr Res 16:111–120, 1995

Beckfield DF: Interpersonal competence among college men hypothesized to be at risk for schizophrenia. J Abnorm Psychol 94:397–404, 1985

Beiser M, Bean G, Erickson D, et al: Biological and psychosocial predictors of job performance following a first episode of psychosis. Am J Psychiatry 151:857–863, 1994

Bellack AS, Morrison RL, Mueser KT, et al: Role-play for assessing the social competence of psychiatric patients. Psychological Assessment 2:248–255, 1990a

Bellack AS, Morrison RL, Wixted JT, et al: An analysis of social competence in schizophrenia. Br J Psychiatry 156:809–818, 1990b

Bellack AS, Mueser KT, Gingerich S, et al: Social Skills Training for Schizophrenia: A Step-By-Step Guide. New York, Guilford, 1997

Bellack AS, Mueser KT, Wade JH, et al: The ability of schizophrenics to perceive and cope with negative affect. Br J Psychiatry 160:473–480, 1992

Bellack AS, Sayers M, Mueser KT, et al: An evaluation of social problem solving in schizophrenia. J Abnorm Psychol 103:371–378, 1994

Benton AL, Hamsher KdeS, Varney NR, et al: Contributions to Neuropsychological Assessment. New York, Oxford University Press, 1983

Berenbaum H, Oltmanns TF: Emotional experience and expression in schizophrenia and depression. J Abnorm Psychol 101:37–44, 1992

Berenbaum H, Snowhite R, Oltmanns TF: Anhedonia and emotional responses to affect evoking stimuli. Psychol Med 17:677–684, 1987

Berman I, Viegner B, Merson A, et al: Differential relationships between positive and negative symptoms and neuropsychological deficits in schizophrenia. Schizophr Res 25:1–10, 1997

Blanchard JJ, Bellack AS, Mueser KT: Affective and social-behavioral correlates of physical and social anhedonia in schizophrenia. J Abnorm Psychol 103:719–728, 1994

Blanchard JJ, Panzarella C: Affect and social functioning in schizophrenia, in Handbook of social functioning in schizophrenia. Edited by Mueser KT, Tarrier N. Needham Heights, MA, Allyn & Bacon, 1998, pp 181–196

Bland RC, Parker JH, Orn H: Prognosis in schizophrenia: a ten-year follow-up of first admissions. Arch Gen Psychiatry 33:949–954, 1976

Bland RC, Parker JH, Orn H: Prognosis in schizophrenia: prognostic predictors and outcome. Arch Gen Psychiatry 35:72–77, 1978

Bleuler E: Dementia Praecox or the Group of Schizophrenias (1911). Translated by Zinkin J. New York, International Universities Press, 1950

Bowen L, Wallace CJ, Glynn SM, et al: Schizophrenic individuals' cognitive functioning and performance in interpersonal interactions and skills training procedures. J Psychiatr Res 28:289–301, 1994

Brandt J: The Hopkins Verbal Learning Test: development of a new memory test with six equivalent forms. The Clinical Neuropsychologist 5:125–142, 1991

Brebion G, Smith MJ, Gorman JM, et al: Reality monitoring failure in schizophrenia: the role of selective attention. Schizophr Res 22:173–180, 1996

Breier A, Schreiber JL, Dyer J, et al: National Institute of Mental Health longitudinal study of chronic schizophrenia: prognosis and predictors of outcome. Arch Gen Psychiatry 48:239–246, 1991

Brekke JS, Raine A, Ansel M, et al: Neuropsychological and psychophysiological correlates of psychosocial functioning in schizophrenia. Schizophr Bull 23:19–28, 1997

Bryson G, Bell M, Lysaker P: Affect recognition in schizophrenia: a function of global impairment or a specific cognitive deficit? Psychiatr Res 71:105–114, 1997

Carpenter WT Jr, Strauss JS: The prediction of schizophrenia, IV: eleven-year follow-up of the Washington IPSS cohort. J Nerv Ment Dis 179:517–525, 1991

Carter M, Flesher S: The neurosociology of schizophrenia: vulnerability and functional disability. Psychiatry 58:209–224, 1995

Chaves AC, Seeman MV, Mari JJ, et al: Schizophrenia: impact of positive symptoms on gender social role. Schizophr Res 11:41–45, 1993

Cohen JD, Servan-Schreiber D: A theory of dopamine function and its role in cognitive deficits in schizophrenia. Schizophr Bull 19:85–104, 1993

Corcoran R, Mercer G, Frith CD: Schizophrenia, symptomatology and social inference: investigating "theory of mind" in people with schizophrenia. Schizophr Res 17:5–13, 1995

Cornblatt BA, Kelip JG: Impaired attention, genetics, and the pathophysiology of schizophrenia. Schizophr Bull 20:31–46, 1994

Cornblatt BA, Lenzenweger MF, Dworkin RH, et al: Childhood attentional dysfunctions predict social deficits in unaffected adults at risk for schizophrenia. Br J Psychiatry Suppl 18:59–64, 1992

Cornblatt B, Obuchowski M, Schnur DB, et al: Attention and clinical symptoms in schizophrenia. Psychiatr Q 68:343–59, 1997

Corrigan PW, Green MF: Schizophrenic patients' sensitivity to social cues: the role of abstraction. Am J Psychiatry 150:589–594, 1993

Corrigan PW, Green MF, Toomey R: Cognitive correlates to social cue perception in schizophrenia. Psychiatry Res 53:141–151, 1994

Corrigan PW, Hirschbeck JN, Wolfe M: Memory and vigilance training to improve social perception in schizophrenia. Schizophr Res 17:257–265, 1995

Corrigan PW, Silverman R, Stephenson J, et al: Situational familiarity and feature recognition in schizophrenia. Schizophr Bull 22:153–161, 1996

Corrigan PW, Wallace CJ, Green MF: Deficits in social schemata in schizophrenia. Schizophr Res 8:129–135, 1992

Corrigan PW, Wallace CJ, Schade ML, et al: Learning medication self-management skills in schizophrenia: Relationships with cognitive deficits and psychiatric symptoms. Behavior Therapy 25:5–15, 1994

Coryell W, Tsuang MT: Outcome after 40 years in DSM-III schizophreniform disorder. Arch Gen Psychiatry 43:324–328, 1986

Crookes TG: A cognitive peculiarity specific to schizophrenia. J Clin Psychol 40:893–896, 1984

Cuesta MJ, Peralta V: Are positive and negative symptoms relevant to cross-sectional diagnosis of schizophrenic and schizoaffective patients? Compr Psychiatry 36:353–361, 1995

Davidson L, McGlashan TH: The varied outcomes of schizophrenia. Can J Psychiatry 42:34–43, 1997

Dawson ME, Nuechterlein KH: Psychophysiological dysfunctions in the developmental course of schizophrenic disorders. Schizophr Bull 10:204–232, 1984

Dickerson F, Boronow JJ, Tringel N, et al: Neurocognitive deficits and social functioning in outpatients with schizophrenia. Schizophr Res 21:75–83, 1996

Dobson DJ, McDougall G, Busheikin J, et al: Effects of social skills training and social milieu treatment on symptoms of schizophrenia. Psychiatr Serv 46:376–380, 1995

Dworkin RH: Affective deficits and social deficits in schizophrenia: what's what? Schizophr Bull 18:59–64, 1992

Eaton WW, Thara R, Federman B, et al: Structure and course of positive and negative symptoms in schizophrenia. Arch Gen Psychiatry 52:127–134, 1995

Elkins IJ, Cromwell RL, Asarnow RF: Span of apprehension in schizophrenic patients as a function of distractor masking and laterality. J Abnorm Psychol 101:53–60, 1992

Erlenmeyer-Kimling L, Cornblatt BA, Rock D, et al: The New York High-Risk Project: anhedonia, attentional deviance, and psychopathology. Schizophr Bull 19:141–153, 1993

Fennig S, Putnam K, Bromet EJ, et al: Gender, premorbid characteristics and negative symptoms in schizophrenia. Acta Psychiatr Scand 92:173–177, 1995

Freedman LR, Rock D, Roberts SA, et al: The New York High-Risk Project: attention, anhedonia and social outcome. Schizophr Res 30:1–9, 1998

Gift TE, Strauss JS, Ritzler BA, et al: Social class and psychiatric outcome. Am J Psychiatry 143:222–225, 1986

Goldman-Rakic PS: Working memory and the mind. Sci Am 267:110–117, 1992

Goldstein JM, Seidman LJ, Goodman JM, et al: Are there sex differences in neuropsychological functions among patients with schizophrenia? Am J Psychiatry 155:1358–1364, 1998

Green MF: What are the functional consequences of neurocognitive deficits in schizophrenia? Am J Psychiatry 153:321–330, 1996

Gupta S, Rajaprabhakaran R, Arndt S, et al: Premorbid adjustment as a predictor of phenomenological and neurobiological indices in schizophrenia. Schizophr Res 16:189–197, 1995

Haberman MC, Chapman LJ, Numbers JS, et al: Relation of social competence to scores on two scales of psychosis proneness. J Abnorm Psychol 88:675–677, 1979

Hafner H, Nowotny B: Epidemiology of early-onset schizophrenia. Eur Arch Psychiatry Clin Neurosci 245:80–92, 1995

Harding CM, Brooks GW, Ashikaga T, et al: The Vermont longitudinal study of persons with severe mental illness, II: long-term outcome of subjects who retrospectively met DSM-III criteria for schizophrenia. Am J Psychiatry 144:727–735, 1987a

Harding CM, Zubin J, Strauss JS: Chronicity in schizophrenia: fact, partial fact, or artifact? Hospital and Community Psychiatry 38:477–486, 1987b

Harris A, Ayers T, Leek ME: Auditory span of apprehension deficits in schizophrenia. J Nerv Ment Dis 173:650–657, 1985

Harrow M, Westermeyer JF, Silverstein M, et al: Predictors of outcome in schizophrenia: the process-reactive dimension. Schizophr Bull 12:195–206, 1986

Harrow M, Yonan CA, Sands JR, et al: Depression in schizophrenia: are neuroleptics, akinesia, or anhedonia involved? Schizophr Bull 20:327–338, 1994

Harvey CA, Curson DA, Pantelis C, et al: Four behavioural syndromes of schizophrenia. Br J Psychiatry 168:562–570, 1996

Harvey PD, Davidson M, Mueser KT, et al: The Social-Adaptive Functioning Evaluation (SAFE): a rating scale for geriatric psychiatric patients. Schizophr Bull 23:131–145, 1997

Heaton RK: The Wisconsin Card Sorting Test. Odessa, FL, Psychological Resources, 1981

Hoffman H, Kupper Z: Relationships between social competence, psychopathology and work performance and their predictive value for vocational rehabilitation of schizophrenic outpatients. Schizophr Res 23:69–79, 1997

Hogarty GE, Flesher S: Cognitive remediation in schizophrenia: proceed...with caution. Schizophr Bull 18:51–57, 1992

Holmes-Eber P, Riger S: Hospitalization and the composition of mental patients' social networks. Schizophr Bull 16:157–164, 1990

Husted JA, Beiser M, Iacono WG: Negative symptoms in the course of first-episode affective psychosis. Psychiatry Res 56:145–154, 1995

Hyde TM, Nawroz S, Goldberg TE, et al: Is there cognitive decline in schizophrenia? A cross-sectional study. Br J Psychiatry 164:494–500, 1994

Ikebuchi E, Nakagome K, Tugawa R, et al: What influences social skills in patients with schizophrenia? preliminary study using the role play test, WAIS-R and event-related potential. Schizophr Res 22:143–150, 1996

Jablensky A, Cole SW: Is the earlier age at onset of schizophrenia in males a confounded finding: results from a cross-cultural investigation. Br J Psychiatry 170:234–240, 1997

Jablensky A, Schwartz R, Tomov T: WHO collaborative study on impairments and disabilities associated with schizophrenic disorders. Acta Psychiatr Scand 62 (suppl 285):152–163, 1980

Jackson HJ, Minas IH, Burgess PM, et al: Is social skills performance a correlate of schizophrenia subtypes? Schizophr Res 2:301–309, 1989

Jaeger J, Douglas E: Neuropsychiatric rehabilitation for persistent mental illness. Psychiatr Q 63:71–74, 1992

Johnstone EC, MacMillan JF, Frith CD, et al: Further investigation of the predictors of outcome following first schizophrenic episodes. Br J Psychiatry 157:182–189, 1990

Jonsson H, Nyman AK: Predicting long-term outcome in schizophrenia. Acta Psychiatr Scand 83:342–346, 1991

Keefe RS, Mohs RC, Losonczy MF, et al: Characteristics of very poor outcome in schizophrenia. Am J Psychiatry 144:889–895, 1987

Keith SJ, Regier DA, Rae DS: Schizophrenic disorders, in Psychiatric Disorders in America: The Epidemiological Catchment Area Study. Edited by Robins LN, Regier DA. New York, Free Press, 1987, pp 33–52

Kelley ME, Gilbertson M, Mouton A, et al: Deterioration in premorbid functioning in schizophrenia: a developmental model of negative symptoms in drug-free patients. Am J Psychiatry 149:1543–1548, 1992

Kern RS, Green MF, Satz P: Neuropsychological predictors of skills training for chronic psychiatric patients. Psychiatry Res 43:223–230, 1992

Kerr SL, Neale JM: Emotion perception in schizophrenia: specific deficit or further evidence of generalized poor performance? J Abnorm Psychol 102:312–318, 1993

Kraepelin E: Dementia Praecox and Paraphrenia (1919). Translated by Barclay RM. Huntingdon, NY, RE Krieger, 1971

Kring AM, Neale JM: Do schizophrenic patients show a disjunctive relationship among expressive, experiential, and psychophysiological components of emotion? J Abnorm Psychol 105:249–257, 1996

Larsen TK, McGlashan TH, Johannessen JO, et al: First-episode schizophrenia, II: premorbid patterns by gender. Schizophr Bull 22:257–269, 1996

Lewine R, Haden C, Caudle J, et al: Sex-onset effects on neuropsychological functioning schizophrenia. Schizophr Bull 23:51–61, 1997

Lezak MD: Neuropsychological Assessment. New York, Oxford University Press, 1976

Liberman RP, DeRisi WJ, Mueser KT: Social Skills Training for Psychiatric Patients. Needham Heights, MA, Allyn & Bacon, 1989

Liberman RP, Mueser KT, Wallace CJ, et al: Training skills in the psychiatrically disabled: learning, coping, and competence. Schizophr Bull 12:631–647, 1986

Lipton FR, Cohen CI, Fischer E, et al: Schizophrenia: a network crisis. Schizophr Bull 7:144–151, 1981

Lysaker P, Bell M: Negative symptoms and vocational impairment in schizophrenia: repeated measurements of work performance over six months. Acta Psychiatr Scand 91:205–208, 1995

Lysaker PH, Bell MD, Bioty SM, et al: The frequency of associations between positive and negative symptoms and dysphoria in schizophrenia. Compr Psychiatry 36:113–117, 1995a

Lysaker PH, Bell MD, Zito WS, et al: Social skills at work: Deficits and predictors of improvement in schizophrenia. J Nerv Ment Dis 183:688–692, 1995b

Marder SR, Wirshing WC, Mintz J, et al: Two-year outcome of social skills training and group psychotherapy for outpatients with schizophrenia. Am J Psychiatry 153:1585–1592, 1996

Marshall M, Hogg LI, Gath DH, et al: The Cardinal Needs Schedule: a modified version of the MRC Needs for Care Assessment Schedule. Psychol Med 25:603–617, 1995

Mason P, Harrison G, Glazebrook C, et al: The course of schizophrenia over 13 years: a report from the International Study on Schizophrenia (ISoS) coordinated by the World Health Organization. Br J Psychiatry 169:580–586, 1996

Massell HK, Corrigan PW, Liberman RP, et al: Conversation skills training of thought-disordered schizophrenic patients through attention focusing. Psychiatry Res 38:51–61, 1991

Maurer K, Bentz C, Loffler W, et al: Seeelische Behinderung–Vorlaufer oder soziale Folge der Schizophrenie? [Psychiatric handicap–precursor or social sequelae of schizophrenia?]. Gesundheitswesen 58 (1 suppl):79–85, 1996

McCreadie RG, Connolly MA, Williamson DJ, et al: The Nithsdale Schizophrenia Surveys, XII: 'neurodevelopmental' schizophrenia: a search for clinical correlates and putative aetiological factors. Br J Psychiatry 65:340–346, 1994

McEvoy JP, Hartman M, Gottlieb D, et al: Common sense, insight, and neuropsychological test performance in schizophrenia patients. Schizophr Bull 22:635–641, 1996

McFall RM: A review and reformulation of the concept of social skills. Behavioral Assessment 4:1–33, 1982

McGlashan TH, Fenton WS: The positive-negative distinction in schizophrenia: review of natural history validators. Arch Gen Psychiatry 49:63–72, 1992

McGlashan TH, Heinssen RK: Hospital discharge status and long-term outcome for patients with schizophrenia, schizoaffective disorder, borderline personality disorder, and unipolar affective disorder. Arch Gen Psychiatry 45:363–368, 1988

McGuffin P, Scourfield J: Human genetics: a father's imprint on his daughter's thinking. Nature 387:652–653, 1997

Meehl PE: Schizotaxia, schizotypy, and schizophrenia. Am Psychol 17:827–838, 1962

Mirsky AF, Duncan CC: Etiology and expression of schizophrenia: neurobiological and psychosocial factors. Annu Rev Psychol 37:291–319, 1986

Mirsky AF, Lochhead SJ, Jones BP, et al: On familial factors in the attentional deficit in schizophrenia: a review and report of two new subject samples. J Psychiatr Res 26:383–403, 1992

Mirsky AF, Yardley SL, Jones BP, et al: Analysis of the attention deficit in schizophrenia: a study of patients and their relatives in Ireland. J Psychiatr Res 29:23–42, 1995

Morice R, Delahunty A: Frontal/executive impairments in schizophrenia. Schizophr Bull 22:125–137, 1996

Morice R: Cognitive inflexibility and pre-frontal dysfunction in schizophrenia and mania. Br J Psychiatry 157:50–54, 1990

Morris RG, Rushe T, Woodruffe PW, et al: Problem solving in schizophrenia: a specific deficit in planning ability. Schizophr Res 14:235–246, 1995

Mueser KT, Bellack AS, Brady EU: Hallucinations in schizophrenia. Acta Psychiatr Scand 82:26–29, 1990a

Mueser KT, Bellack AS, Morrison RL, et al: Gender, social competence, and symptomatology in schizophrenia: a longitudinal analysis. J Abnorm Psychol 99:138–147, 1990b

Mueser KT, Bellack AS, Morrison RL, et al: Social competence in schizophrenia: premorbid adjustment, social skill, and domains of functioning. J Psychiatr Res 24:51–63, 1990c

Mueser KT, Bellack AS, Douglas MS, et al: Prediction of social skill acquisition in schizophrenic and major affective disorder patients from memory and symptomatology. Psychiatry Res 37:281–296, 1991a

Mueser KT, Bellack AS, Douglas MS, et al: Prevalence and stability of social skill deficits in schizophrenia. Schizophr Res 5:167–176, 1991b

Mueser KT, Douglas MS, Bellack AS, et al: Assessment of enduring deficit and negative symptom subtypes in schizophrenia. Schizophr Bull 17:565–582, 1991c

Mueser KT, Blanchard JJ, Bellack AS: Memory and social skill in schizophrenia: the role of gender. Psychiatry Res 57:141–153, 1995

Mueser KT, Doonan R, Penn DL, et al: Emotion recognition and social competence in chronic schizophrenia. J Abnorm Psychol 105:271–275, 1996

Mueser KT, Becker DR, Torrey WC, et al: Work and nonvocational domains of functioning in persons with severe mental illness: a longitudinal analysis. J Nerv Ment Dis 185:419–426, 1997

Munroe-Blum H, Collins E, McCleary L, et al: The Social Dysfunction Index (SDI) for patients with schizophrenia and related disorders. Schizophr Res 20:211–219, 1996

Neumann CS, Grimes K, Walker EF, et al: Developmental pathways to schizophrenia: behavioral subtypes. J Abnorm Psychol 104:558–566, 1995

Niwa S-I, Hiramatsu K-I, Saitoh O, et al: Information dysregulation and event-related potentials in schizophrenia. Schizophr Bull 18:95–105, 1992

Nuechterlein KH, Dawson ME: Information processing and attentional functioning in the developmental course of schizophrenic disorders. Schizophr Bull 10:160–203, 1984

Nuechterlein KH, Edell WS, Norris M, et al: Attentional vulnerability indicators, thought disorder, and negative symptoms. Schizophr Bull 12:408–426, 1986

Numbers JS, Chapman LJ: Social deficits in hypothetically psychosis-prone college women. J Abnorm Psychol 91:255–260, 1982

Odegaard O: Marriage and mental disease: a study in social psychopathology. Journal of Mental Science 92:35–59, 1946

Odegaard O: The incidence of psychoses in various occupations. International Journal of Social Psychiatry 2:85–104, 1956

Odegaard O: Marriage rates and fertility in psychotic patients before hospital admission and after discharge. International Journal of Social Psychiatry 6:25–33, 1960

Osterrieth PA: Le test de copie d'une figure complexe. Archives de Psychologie 30:206–356, 1944

Penn DL, Mueser KT: Research update on the psychosocial treatment of schizophrenia. Am J Psychiatry 153:607–617, 1996

Penn DL, van der Does W, Spaulding W, et al: Information processing and social cognitive problem solving in schizophrenia. J Nerv Ment Dis 191:13–20, 1993

Penn DL, Hope DA, Spaulding W, et al: Social anxiety in schizophrenia. Schizophr Res 11:277–284, 1994

Penn DL, Mueser KT, Doonan R, et al: Relations between social skills and ward behavior in chronic schizophrenia. Schizophr Res 16:225–232, 1995a

Penn DL, Mueser KT, Spaulding W, et al: Information processing and social competence in chronic schizophrenia. Schizophr Bull 21:269–281, 1995b

Penn DL, Mueser KT, Spaulding W: Information processing, social skill, and gender in schizophrenia. Psychiatry Res 59:213–220, 1996

Penn DL, Corrigan PW, Bentall RP, et al: Social cognition in schizophrenia. Psychol Bull 121:114–132, 1997

Peralta V, Cuesta MJ, deLeon J: Positive and negative symptoms/syndromes in schizophrenia: reliability and validity of different diagnostic systems. Psychol Med 25:43–50, 1995

Perlick D, Stastny P, Mattis S, et al: Contribution of family, cognitive, and clinical dimensions to long-term outcome in schizophrenia. Schizophr Res 6:257–265, 1992

Perry W, Moore D, Braff D: Gender differences on though disturbance measures among schizophrenic patients. Am J Psychiatry 152:1298–1301, 1995

Pescolido BA: Illness careers and network ties: a conceptual model of utilization and compliance. Advances in Medical Sociology 2:161–184, 1991

Pogue-Geile MF, Harrow M: Negative and positive symptoms in schizophrenia and depression: a follow up. Schizophr Bull 10:371–387, 1984

Pogue-Geile MF: The prognostic significance of negative symptoms in schizophrenia. Br J Psychiatry Suppl 7:123–127, 1989

Reitan RM: The Halstead-Reitan Neuropsychological Battery: Theory and Clinical Practice. Tucson, AZ, Neuropsychology Press, 1985

Rey A: L'examen psychologique dans les cas d'encephalopathie traumatique. Archives de Psychologie 28:286–340, 1942

Robins E, Guze SB: Establishment of diagnostic validity in psychiatric illness: its application to schizophrenia. Am J Psychiatry 126:983–987, 1970

Robins LN, Locke BZ, Regier DA: An overview of psychiatric disorders in America, in Psychiatric Disorders in America: The Epidemiological Catchment Area Study. Edited by Robins LN, Regier DA. New York, Free Press, 1991, pp 328–336

Roy MA, DeVriendt X: Positive and negative symptoms in schizophrenia: a current overview. Can J Psychiatry 39:407–414, 1994

Rund BR: Fully recovered schizophrenics: a retrospective study of some premorbid and treatment factors. Psychiatry 53:127–139, 1990

Rund BR, Torgelsboen AK: Fully recovered schizophrenics compared to chronic patients on premorbid and treatment characteristics. Psychiatry and Psychobiology 5:113–121, 1990

Salokangas RK, Rakkolainen V, Alanen YO: Maintenance of grip on life and goals of life: a valuable criterion for evaluating outcome in schizophrenia. Acta Psychiatr Scand 80:187–193, 1989

Sayers SL, Curran PJ, Mueser KT: Factor structure and construct validity of the scale for the assessment of negative symptoms. Psychological Assessment 8:269–280, 1996

Schmidt M, Blanz B, Dippe A, et al: Course of patients diagnosed as having schizophrenia during first episode occurring under age 18 years. Eur Arch Psychiatry Clin Neurosci 245:93–100, 1995

Schooler N, Hogarty G, Weissman M: Social Adjustment Scale II (SAS-II), in Resource Materials for Community Mental Health Program Evaluations (DHEW Publication No. (ADM) 79-328). Edited by Hargreaves WA, Atkisson CC, Sorenson JE. Rockville, MD, National Institute of Mental Health, 1978

Scott JE, Lehman AF: Social functioning in the community, in Handbook of Social Functioning in Schizophrenia. Edited by Mueser KT, Tarrier N. Needham Heights, MA, Allyn & Bacon, 1998, pp 1–19

Shallice T: Specific impairments of planning. Philos Trans R Soc Lond B Biol Sci 298:199–209, 1982

Shankar R, Kamath S, Joseph AA: Gender differences in disability: a comparison of married patients with schizophrenia. Schizophr Res 16:17–23, 1995

Skuse DH, James RS, Bishop DV, et al: Evidence from Turner's syndrome of an imprinted X-linked locus affecting cognitive function. Nature 387:705–708, 1997

Smith TE, Hull JW, Anthony DT, et al: Post-hospitalization treatment adherence of schizophrenic patients: gender differences in skill acquisition. Psychiatry Res 69:123–129, 1997

Solinski S, Jackson HJ, Bell RC: Prediction of employability in schizophrenic patients. Schizophr Res 7:141–148, 1992

Spaulding WD, Storms L, Goodrich V, et al: Applications of experimental psychopathology in psychiatric rehabilitation. Schizophr Bull 12:560–577, 1986

Stein J: Vocal alterations in schizophrenic speech. J Nerv Ment Dis 181:59–62, 1993

Stirling JD, Hellewell JSE, Hewitt J: Verbal memory impairment in schizophrenia: no sparing of short-term recall. Schizophr Res 25:85–95, 1997

Strauss JS, Carpenter WT Jr: The prediction of outcome in schizophrenia, I: characteristics of outcome. Arch Gen Psychiatry 27:739–746, 1972

Strauss JS, Carpenter WT Jr: The prediction of outcome in schizophrenia, II: relationships between predictor and outcome variables. A report from the WHO International Pilot Study of Schizophrenia. Arch Gen Psychiatry 31:37–42, 1974

Strauss JS, Carpenter WT Jr: Prediction of outcome in schizophrenia, III: five-year outcome and its predictors. Arch Gen Psychiatry 27:739–746, 1977

Stroop JR: Studies of interference in serial verbal reactions. Journal of Experimental Psychology 18:643–662, 1935

Sullivan G, Marder SR, Liberman RP, et al: Social skills and relapse history in outpatient schizophrenics. Psychiatry 53:340–345, 1990

Tessler RC, Manderscheid RW: Factors affecting adjustment to community living. Hospital and Community Psychiatry 33:203–207, 1982

Tsuang MT: Memory deficit and long-term outcome in schizophrenia: a preliminary study. Psychiatry Res 6:355–360, 1982

van den Bosch RJ, Rombouts RP, van Asma MJ: What determines continuous performance task performance? Schizophr Bull 22:643–651, 1996

Vazquez-Barquero JL, Cuesta Nunez MJ, Herrera Castanedo S, et al: Sociodemographic and clinical variables as predictors of the diagnostic characteristics of first episodes of schizophrenia. Acta Psychiatr Scand 94:149–55, 1996

Velligan DE, Mahurin RK, Eckert SL, et al: Relationship between specific types of communication deviance and attentional performance in patients with schizophrenia. Psychiatry Res 70:9–20, 1997

Verdoux H, van Os J, Sham P, et al: Does familiality predispose to both emergence and persistence of psychosis? a follow-up study. Br J Psychiatry 168:620–626, 1996

Wallace CJ, Nelson CJ, Liberman RP, et al: A review and critique of social skills training with schizophrenic patients. Schizophr Bull 6:42–63, 1980

Weintraub S: Risk factors in schizophrenia: the Stony Brook High-Risk Project. Schizophr Bull 13:439–450, 1987

Wykes T, Sturt E: The measurement of social behaviour in psychiatric patients: an assessment of the reliability and validity of the SBS Schedule. Br J Psychiatry 148:1–11, 1986

Wykes T, Sturt E, Katz R: The prediction of rehabilitative success after three years: the use of social, symptom, and cognitive variables. Br J Psychiatry 157:865–877, 1990

Yang PC, Liu CY, Chiang SQ, et al: Comparison of adult manifestations of schizophrenia with onset before and after 15 years of age. Acta Psychiatr Scand 91:209–212, 1995

Young DA, Freyslinger MG: Scaffolded instruction and the remediation of Wisconsin Card Sorting Test deficits in chronic schizophrenia. Schizophr Res 16:199–207, 1995

Wechsler D: Wechsler Adult Intelligence Scale–Revised. San Antonio, TX, Psychological Corporation, 1981

Wechsler D: Wechsler Memory Scale–Revised. San Antonio, TX, Psychological Corporation, 1987

4 Evaluation of Negative Symptoms in Short-Term Pharmacological Trials

Jean-Pierre Lindenmayer, M.D.

There has been renewed recognition of and emphasis on the central position of negative symptoms in schizophrenia. Although this separate psychopathological domain was long ago recognized by Kraepelin (1919/1971), who described the symptoms as "the weakening of these emotional activities which permanently form the mainspring of volition," negative symptoms have been rediscovered in the last 10 years as a result of biological research for more homogeneous subgroups of schizophrenic patients and the development of newer pharmacological compounds with possible effects on negative symptoms. The pathophysiological and etiological mechanisms underlying negative symptoms are most likely different from those underlying positive symptoms. Beyond their importance as representing an identifiable symptom group (or *syndrome*) within the heterogeneity of schizophrenic symptoms, negative symptoms may also have a more specific association with cognitive deficits, abnormal involuntary movements, and poor social functioning. Hence, the ability to reliably recognize these symptoms and to assess their extent and response to treatment interventions is equally important for clinicians and researchers.

As pharmacotherapy of schizophrenia has evolved and new compounds have been developed, the amelioration of negative symptoms has become one of the new frontiers of schizophrenia. Novel antipsychotic agents·such as risperidone (Marder and Meibach 1994), olanzapine (Tollefson et al. 1996), sertindole (Zimbroff et al. 1997), and quetiapine (Rak and Arvanitis 1997) have been reported to have various amounts of superior efficacy on negative symptoms in comparison with placebo or conventional neuroleptics (usually haloperidol). All of these reports have been based on results from short-term multicenter clinical trials conducted in a variety of schizophrenic patient groups. In this chapter, I will review the evaluation of negative symptoms in such trials and the assessment procedures employed, which are usually based on symptom rating scales specifically developed to enable the researcher to measure negative symptoms and their response to treatment.

Measurement of Negative Symptoms

Although there is overall agreement on the existence of a semi-independent negative symptom domain (or negative syndrome) within the schizophrenic psychopathological presentation, there is little agreement about which symptoms are distinctively negative. In a review of methods for measuring negative symptoms, Fenton and McGlashan (1992) compared seven rating scales with regard to the types of symptoms included. In descending order of frequency, the following symptoms appeared in the seven scales: 1) affective flattening, 2) unchanging expression, 3) affective nonresponsivity, 4) lack of vocal inflection, 5) poverty of speech, 6) poverty of content of speech, 7) anhedonia/asociality, 8) emotional withdrawal, 9) psychomotor retardation, and 10) lack of sense of purpose. Each of these 10 symptoms was included in at least two of the seven rating scales, reflecting a moderate degree of agreement among the scales.

There is also disagreement on how best to measure the intensity of each symptom. General requirements for the reliable measurement of negative symptoms are as follows.

The content of a scale—that is, the item selection—is of crucial importance. A key principle for establishing good content validity is adequate representation of each facet of the construct (Nunnally 1978). Thus, if a scale sets out to assess negative symptoms, it must sample manifestations from different functional spheres that are presumed to be involved in the negative symptom construct. The choice of negative items should reflect the underlying construct of *primary* negative features—that is, the inclusion of *secondary* manifestations of negative symptoms should be avoided. For example, poor attention is usually a correlate of positive symptoms and should not be included as a negative symptom. Other frequent confounds, such as depression, extrapyramidal side effects (EPS), and psychosis, must also be separated from negative symptoms (Carpenter et al. 1988). In addition, it is crucial that a measure of overall psychopathology be included in the scale, because negative symptoms covary strongly with global severity of illness (Kay et al. 1986). Furthermore, the intensity range of each item should cover a sufficient number of severity degrees to permit maximal sensitivity.

A second principle of content validity is the inclusion of a relatively large number of items, since this helps to cancel out random error variance, thereby improving reliability. It is also desirable that the major subscales, both positive and negative, contain similar numbers of items, so that their potential reliabilities are comparable. Symptom definitions need to be operationalized and should include detailed criteria for levels of symptom severity. The specific basis for rating (e.g., patient interview vs. staff) and the duration of time over which symptoms are to be assessed must be defined. The validity of the assessment can be compromised if raters use different sources of information about the patient. After the scale is constructed, studies should ascertain its psychometric properties in terms of interrater reliability, test–retest reliability, internal consistency, and content and construct validity. It should be noted that few of the scales listed below fulfill these requirements.

1. *Scale for the Assessment of Negative Symptoms* (SANS; Andreasen 1982; Andreasen and Olsen 1982): Andreasen pioneered the measurement of well-defined symptoms as captured in five global domains: affective flattening, alogia, avolition/apathy, anhedonia/asociality, and attentional impairment. Each of these global areas is rated further on specific signs on a scale of 1 (not at all) to 5 (severe). A major problem with the SANS is the admittance of attentional impairment as a negative symptom. This symptom correlates highly with positive symptoms (Bilder et al. 1985; Kay et al. 1986) and therefore should probably not have been included.

2. *Positive and Negative Syndrome Scale* (PANSS; Kay et al. 1987): The PANSS is a 30-item, seven-point rating system that was specifically developed to measure positive, negative and other symptom dimensions in schizophrenia (Kay et al. 1987). The PANSS items were selected according to Crow's positive–negative concept (Crow 1980). After a structured clinical interview (SCI-PANSS), a positive and a negative subscale are each assessed as the sum of 7 items, each rated on a severity scale ranging from 1 ("absent") to 7 ("extreme psychopathology"). The 7 negative items comprise the negative subscale: Blunted Affect, Emotional Withdrawal, Poor Rapport, Passive/Apathetic Social Withdrawal, Difficulty in Abstract Thinking, Lack of Spontaneity and Flow of Conversation, and Stereotyped Thinking. The sum of another 16 items that cannot definitively be classified as positive or negative serves as a subscale of general psychopathology. Each item is fully operationalized, and the degrees of severity (1–7) are specifically anchored with a clinical descriptor for each item. The PANSS has shown good

psychometric properties (Lindenmayer 1997) and sensitivity to change. It is particularly useful in tracking negative symptoms over time in response to pharmacological interventions.

3. *Krawiecka-Manchester Scale* (Krawiecka et al. 1977): Only eight items are included in this scale, which was specifically designed not to measure the negative symptom construct but rather to serve as a screening instrument for large psychotic populations. Of these eight items, only four measure negative symptoms: poverty of speech, flat affect, incongruous affect, and psychomotor retardation. The item composition of the Krawiecka-Manchester Scale was modified by Johnstone et al. (1978) and Crow (1985), who removed "incongruous affect" and "psychomotor retardation," leaving only two negative symptoms—poverty of speech and flat affect. These changes reduced the scale's relevancy for negative symptoms.

4. *Scale for Emotional Blunting* (Abrams and Taylor 1978): This rating scale has an adequate sampling of 12 negative symptoms reflecting the underlying construct. However, the items are not operationalized, and the scoring range is only 0–2, thus limiting the scale's sensitivity to change.

5. *Negative Symptom Rating Scale* (NSRS; Iager et al. 1985): The NSRS includes 10 negative symptoms scored on an adequate range of 0–6; however, 3 of these symptoms (memory, attention, and judgment/decision) cannot be clearly related to either a negative or a positive construct. Although items are well operationalized and levels of severity are anchored, the scale includes no comparative assessment of general psychopathology and positive features.

6. *Negative Symptom Scale* (Lewine et al. 1983): The 10 items chosen for this scale have been excerpted from the Schedule for Affective Disorders and Schizophrenia–Change Version (SADS-C; Endicott and Spitzer 1978) and cover some aspects of that scale's four-negative-symptom construct. However, a number of the items, such as fatigue, depressed appearance, loose associations, and incoherence, either are not separable from positive symptoms or relate to neither the positive nor the negative symptom construct.

7. *Schedule for the Deficit Syndrome* (SDS; Kirkpatrick et al. 1989): The criteria for the deficit syndrome require the enduring presence of at least two of a total of six negative symptoms that are considered primary manifestations of the illness (Kirkpatrick et al. 1992). The negative symptoms must have persisted for a minimum of 12 months. Clearly, this scale is designed not for measuring the quantity and change of negative symp-

toms, but rather for classifying patients into deficit/nondeficit categories. Assignment of patients to the deficit group identifies them as having a fixed trait of "deficit" which, by definition, is not sensitive to treatment or course evolution. Thus, use of the SDS is appropriate only for ensuring a certain homogeneity within a subgroup of schizophrenic patients in studies examining specific underlying pathophysiological or neurostructural mechanisms of the negative syndrome.

Despite their inclusion of different negative items, all seven negative symptom scales were found to be highly correlated as dimensional systems when used by Fenton and McGlashan (1992) in the assessment of 187 schizophrenia patients, a result that supports the notion of the negative syndrome construct.

A major theoretical problem that is only partially resolved in most of these rating scales is the distinction between primary and secondary negative symptoms. Carpenter and Buchanan (1989) have highlighted the need to differentiate between primary, "enduring" negative symptoms and secondary negative symptoms due to medication effects, depression, anxiety, or environmental deprivation, as assessed with their instrument, the SDS. In addition, patients who are classified as having the deficit syndrome must have had their negative symptoms for at least 1 year. Consequently, Carpenter asserts that "substantiating claims for [efficacious pharmacotherapy of primary negative symptoms] requires distinguishing primary from secondary negative symptoms and showing that any such drug effect is independent of antipsychotic action" (Carpenter 1992, p. 237). The requirement that negative symptoms persist for a year renders these symptoms virtually immutable and pharmacologically resistant to treatment. Treatments to be tested with this paradigm are almost a priori destined to fail. Carpenter's deficit concept is, therefore, an unsuitable model on which to base measurements of the efficacy of different treatments for negative symptoms.

On the other hand, as stated above, a number of these scales (e.g., the PANSS, the SANS) have taken pains to include as negative items only negative symptoms that are primary in nature. Specifically, factor analytic studies have supported the independence of negative symptoms from depression and positive symptoms as measured by the PANSS (Lindenmayer and Kay 1989). Furthermore, statistical procedures can be used, as described in the following section, to examine the relationship of negative symptom change to other possible etiological sources (e.g., EPS change).

For the clinician, the effect of a particular new treatment on the combination of primary and secondary negative symptoms may be more important than the treatment's differential effect on primary versus secondary symptoms. For those "who wish to relieve the group of negative symptoms…sorting out primary versus secondary issues may be less important than providing assistance in the recovery of normal function" (Meltzer et al. 1991).

Strategies for the Assessment of Change in Negative Symptoms

Establishing Specific Criteria for Patient Inclusion and Study Duration

An important strategy for the assessment of negative symptom change is the selection of patients who present with high negative symptom and low positive symptom scores at baseline. Meltzer et al. (1991) reported on 20 neuroleptic-resistant patients with high negative and low positive symptoms and 16 patients with high negative and high positive symptoms treated for 6 months with clozapine. The median improvement in negative symptoms in these patients was 40% after adjustment for changes in ratings of EPS and depression. Two good design features were combined in this study. The first of these features—selection of a patient sample with high negative and low positive symptoms that did not change during the trial—eliminated the possibility of a direct effect of positive symptom change on negative symptom change. The second feature—the extended length of time used to observe change in negative symptoms—allowed a more accurate assessment of treatment effects on primary negative symptoms. This second feature relates to the time frame necessary for change in primary negative symptoms. It is probable that the underlying pathophysiological mechanisms of primary negative symptoms need an extended time frame to respond to pharmacological intervention. Therefore, short-term pharmacological studies more likely will measure treatment effects on the combination of positive and negative symptoms, whereas longer-lasting studies (6–12 months) will measure predominantly primary negative symptoms.

Demonstrating Negative Symptom Effects in the Absence of Positive Symptom Effects

The specific pharmacotherapeutic response of negative symptoms can also be demonstrated when the particular compound under study has no effect on positive symptoms. One such study was conducted by Heresco-Levy et al.

(1996), who examined the effect on both negative and positive symptoms of adding glycine to a stable antipsychotic regimen. Eleven treatment-resistant patients with chronic schizophrenia completed this double-blind, placebo-controlled, 6-week crossover trial of adjuvant glycine therapy. All patients showed stable pretreatment baselines without change in PANSS scores during the 2 weeks prior to randomization. Patients receiving glycine addition showed a significant decrease in PANSS negative symptoms (37.0 to 24.4; $F = 42.5$; $P < .0001$). Positive symptoms did not change significantly (24.6 to 21.0) over this 6-week trial. No change in EPS was observed. The effect of glycine on negative symptoms remained significant after correcting for the effects of changes in cognitive symptoms or depression ($F = 6.8$; $P < .032$), pointing to a marked decrease in primary negative symptoms without change in psychosis or extrapyramidal symptoms.

Although the use of study designs that specifically select patients with high scores on negative symptoms or that examine compounds with exclusive anti–negative symptom action are needed, new antipsychotic compounds may have simultaneous antipsychotic and antinegative effects. These compounds are most often tested initially in patients with acute exacerbations of psychosis–a population in which the differential diagnosis of negative symptoms is notoriously difficult. In the following section, I review a number of statistical procedures that have been used to tease out negative symptom change from other possible mediating change processes in these trials.

Using Statistical Correction

Among the various statistical strategies for assessing negative symptom change, three have been most frequently used to elucidate the relationship of negative symptom change with other possible mediating processes.

Correlational Analysis

This procedure was used by Miller et al. (1994) in a study examining the response of negative symptoms to clozapine. In this 6-week uncontrolled trial with 29 treatment-resistant patients, improvements in negative, psychotic, and disorganization factors, as measured by the Scale for the Assessment of Positive Symptoms (SAPS; Andreasen 1984) and the SANS, were found. A significant improvement was also reported for EPS. Although these change scores were all correlated with negative symptom change, only the correlation of negative-factor change with disorganization-factor change was statistically significant ($r = .52$, $P < .01$). These results point to the relative independence of negative symptom change from positive symptom change but also to some relationship between improvement in negative symptoms and improvement in disorganization symptoms. While this relationship does not imply causality, it nonetheless brings up two questions: 1) Did negative symptoms improve parallel to and independent from disorganization symptoms? and 2) Did improvement in disorganization symptoms (e.g., formal thought disorder or poverty of content of speech) mediate the improvement in negative symptoms? Given the simultaneous presence of negative and disorganization symptoms in these patients, these questions cannot be fully answered with the present design. Correlational analysis thus provides limited further insights on the nature of negative symptom change.

Multiple Regression Analysis

To determine whether other secondary causes are contributing to the improvement in negative symptoms, these secondary factors can be entered into stepwise multiple regression models. Models can examine whether baseline negative symptom ratings or changes in psychotic symptoms or EPS can predict the final negative symptom ratings. In the study by Miller et al. (1994), the baseline negative symptom score was the only significant predictor of the negative symptom rating at endpoint ($F = 10.2$; $P = .004$) after other possible confounding factors—such as change in psychotic symptoms or in EPS—were accounted for.

Analysis of Covariance

Analysis of covariance can be used to compare improvements in negative symptoms in different treatment groups of a pharmacological trial while controlling for the effects of possible confounds, such as change in positive symptoms or in EPS. An analysis of this type of was conducted with the PANSS and the Extrapyramidal Symptom Rating Scale (ESRS; Chouinard et al. 1980) data in the North American risperidone study (Chouinard et al. 1993; Marder and Meibach 1994). In that study, a total of 523 patients with DSM-III-R (American Psychiatric Association 1987) diagnoses of schizophrenia were randomized to 1) one of four different dosages of risperidone (2, 6, 10, or 16 mg/day), 2) haloperidol at 20 mg/day, or 3) placebo. Patients were treated for 8 weeks, and outcomes were assessed with the PANSS. Statistically significant differences relative to placebo were seen in positive symptoms in response to the 6-mg, 10-mg, and 16-mg daily dosages of risperidone and in response to the 20-mg daily dose of haloperidol. PANSS negative symptom scores were significantly reduced compared with placebo in patients receiving the 6 mg and 16 mg risperidone doses, whereas EPS were higher in patients treated with 16 mg of risperidone or 20 mg of haloperidol. The level of EPS in patients receiving 6 mg/day of risperidone was no higher than that in the placebo group. The question that arose was whether the improvement in negative symptoms seen in patients receiving 6 mg/day of risperidone was mediated by risperidone's low level of EPS. To address this question, our group (J. P. Lindenmayer and S. R. Kay, unpublished) conducted an analysis of covariance on the endpoint PANSS negative symptom change with change in ESRS total symptom change as covariate. The results indicated that the change in negative symptoms in patients treated with 6 mg ($P <$ .0001), 10 mg ($P <$ .03), and 16 mg ($P <$ .001) of risperidone remained significant compared with placebo treatment, while the 2-mg risperidone group and the haloperidol group showed no difference from placebo-treated patients. This finding is even further strengthened by the observation that patients receiving 16 mg/day of risperidone showed improvement in negative symptoms despite having the highest level of EPS of any of the risperidone groups. These results support the ability of the PANSS to differentiate between negative symptoms and EPS in acute schizophrenic patients treated with pharmacological agents.

Path Analysis

Möller et al. (1995) have proposed the use of path analysis to differentiate between indirect and direct effects. This technique allows a drug's direct effects on certain symptoms to be assessed by separating those effects from the drug's indirect effects on other symptoms. Path analysis has been applied in trials with atypical antipsychotics to examine the effect of these agents on negative symptoms while correcting for confounding effects from baseline negative symptoms, positive symptoms, depression, and EPS. In two such trials (R. Tandon, C. Silber, and R. Mack, presentation at the 10th Congress of the European College of Neuropsychopharmacology, Vienna, Austria, 13–17 September 1997), 497 and 462 schizophrenic patients were randomized in two different studies examining the efficacy of sertindole (M93-113 and M93-O98) to 12, 20, or 24 mg of sertindole and compared with 4, 8, and 16 mg of haloperidol. The path analysis revealed that sertindole's direct effect on PANSS negative symptoms was significantly greater than that of haloperidol. Thus, the use of this technique allowed investigators to separate sertindole's direct effects on negative symptoms from its indirect effects on those symptoms via reduction in EPS (since sertindole has a lower propensity to cause EPS than does haloperidol).

Factor Analysis

Another useful strategy for examining change in negative symptoms is factor analysis, an approach that uses rating scales measuring a wide spectrum of psychopathology to identify semi-independent but coexisting domains of psychopathology. Lindenmayer (1993) conducted a principal components analysis in 517 DSM-III-R-diagnosed schizophrenia inpatients who were part of the North American risperidone study. Factor analysis of the patients' baseline PANSS scores yielded five symptom domains explaining 56.2% of the variance: negative, positive, cognitive, excitement, and depression/anxiety. Examination of the correlations among these items revealed that whereas the negative and depression/anxiety items were independent, the negative and cognitive items were significantly correlated at .3 ($P < .03$).

Clinical Implications

The issues involved in the assessment of negative symptoms are different for clinicians than for researchers. Historically, the positive symptoms of schizophrenia—delusions, hallucinations, and disorganized behavior—were emphasized. Patients with predominantly negative symptoms were less likely to be brought to the attention of a treating clinician, perhaps because such patients were not seen as presenting management problems. The first challenge for clinicians is to learn to recognize negative symptoms in their patients. Clinicians must therefore elevate their recognition threshold for negative symptoms and recognize that many of these symptoms are amenable to pharmacological treatment. One way to increase awareness of these symptoms' presence in patients is to use a validated rating scale. Ideally, clinicians could include one of the assessment instruments described above in their routine clinical evaluations of schizophrenic patients.

In addition, some shorter clinical assessment instruments have been introduced that can be administered either by the treating psychiatrist or by other trained mental health professionals working with the patient. One such instrument is the Negative Symptom Assessment (Chiles et al. 1999). This measure was developed as part of the Texas Medication Algorithm—Schizophrenia Module (Chiles et al. 1999) and consists of four questions that are rated by the examiner on a four-point scale. This short assessment tool has shown good correlation with assessments conducted with more formal negative symptom scales. Another instrument, the Psychosis Evaluation tool for Common use by Caregivers (PECC), was derived from the PANSS (Kay et al. 1989) and has been modified by De Hert et al. (1999). It contains most of the PANSS items, clustered into five syndromal domains, one of which is a negative syndrome domain, as proposed originally by Lindenmayer et al. (1995). The severity levels (1–7) of each item have been simplified and four new items have been added. Both of these shorter instruments can easily be used as follow-up and outcome measures in routine psychopharmacological inpatient and outpatient treatment of schizophrenic patients.

More clinically oriented clues as to the presence and extent of negative symptoms are summarized in the guidelines provided below.

1. Base the assessment of negative symptoms on the interview with the patient and the reports of significant others and of the nursing staff in order to obtain information on the patient's social interactions, initiatives, degree of speech output, and quality of interactions. Use multiple sources of information.

2. Observe the patient's facial expression during the course of the interview, the degree of his or her use of gestures to support conversation, and the facial response to a humorous intervention by the clinician.

3. Conduct an examination of the extrapyramidal system to diagnose akinesia and bradykinesia, which can confound negative symptoms.

4. Determine whether depression, demoralization, and/ anhedonia, which also can overlap with negative symptoms, are present.

5. Assess the speech latency and verbal output of the patient in his or her responses to questions by the interviewer. Patients with significant negative symptoms will take considerable time to answer questions, and the overall verbal output will be impoverished. Similarly, patients' overall reaction time will be prolonged in the presence of significant negative symptoms.

These guidelines are demonstrated in the following clinical example.

Mr. F, a 36-year-old single man, has a long history of psychiatric admissions over the past 15 years and a diagnosis of schizophrenia, chronic undifferentiated type. He was discharged 4 months ago to the local community mental health center after a 3-week admission due to psychotic decompensation following his noncompliance with antipsychotic medication. He was restabilized on an intramuscular depot antipsychotic regimen, which he tolerates well without significant EPS. At present, Mr. F attends the day program at the community mental health center, lives in a supervised residence, and has minimal contacts with his family. He denies delusional thinking, shows a mild thought disorder, and complains of occasional auditory hallucinations, which, however, do not interfere with his day-to-day functioning. At the center, Mr. F is observed to have minimal contacts with his peers and to lack initiative. He is clearly detached from persons and events in the milieu, although he is docile and will attend group activities on prompting, but with little active participation. When asked why he is not more involved, Mr. F answers that he is not interested in the program. In response to questions about current political events, he shows only moderate awareness of what is going on in the world, despite the fact that he watches television at the center whenever there are no activities scheduled. Mr. F tends to his personal needs but is somewhat neglectful of his attire. He has no friends in the center despite the fact that he spent time there after his previous discharges. In one-on-one conversation, his verbal output is limited and he avoids direct eye contact. Mr. F denies feelings of depression or demoralization; he states that, overall, he likes the center.

Mr. F demonstrates clear negative symptoms that have been stable for the past 4 months. There is no significant contribution from EPS or depression. Mr. F is enrolled in an active program with disease-specific activities. He is eventually switched from his typical antipsychotic medication to an atypical one and shows a partial response in his negative symptoms. Mr. F becomes more involved during group meetings, his verbal output increases, and he no longer avoids direct eye contact. Although his occasional auditory hallucinations remain, Mr. F's level of interaction clearly increases.

Conclusions

Negative schizophrenic symptoms can be measured in a reliable and valid manner with a number of rating scales. The choice of a particular rating scale depends on the specific aims of the study at hand. Scales such as the SANS and the PANSS have succeeded to some extent in measuring primary negative symptoms separate from depression, positive symptoms, and EPS confounds. However, distinguishing between primary and secondary negative symptoms is very difficult, especially during an acute psychotic phase, when the two domains of psychopathology often coexist. Change in negative symptoms can be measured through the use of appropriate study designs or by applying specific statistical procedures to reduce the influence of the effects of other processes, such as EPS, positive symptoms, and depression. Although these procedures allow for a satisfactory assessment of change under different pharmacological conditions, new techniques that quantify "negative" behaviors—such as analyses of vocal acoustics (Knight and Roff 1985), ratings of facial movements (Andreasen et al. 1981), and measures of speech quantity and rate (Alpert 1983)—must be explored further in order to achieve greater specificity in the assessment of negative symptoms.

References

Abrams R, Taylor MA: A rating scale for emotional blunting. Am J Psychiatry 135:226–229, 1978

Alpert M: Encoding of feelings and voice, in Treatment of Depression: Old Controversies and New Approaches. Edited by Clayton PJ, Barret JE. New York, Raven, 1983

American Psychiatric Association: Diagnostic and Statistical Manual of Mental Disorders, 3rd Edition, Revised. Washington, DC, American Psychiatric Association, 1987

Andreasen NC: Negative symptoms in schizophrenia: definition and reliability. Arch Gen Psychiatry 39:784–788, 1982

Andreasen NC: The Scale for the Assessment of Positive Symptoms (SAPS). Iowa City, University of Iowa, 1984

Andreasen NC, Olsen SA: Negative vs. positive schizophrenia: definition and validation. Arch Gen Psychiatry 39:789–794, 1982

Andreasen NC, Alpert MK, Martz MJ: Acoustic analysis: an objective measure of affective flattening. Arch Gen Psychiatry 38:281–285, 1981

Bilder RM, Mukherjee S, Reider RO, et al: Symptomatic and neuropsychological components of defect states. Schizophr Bull 11:409–419, 1985

Carpenter WT Jr: The negative symptom challenge. Arch Gen Psychiatry 49:236–237, 1992

Carpenter WT Jr, Buchanan RW: Domains of psychopathology relevant to the study of etiology and treatment of schizophrenia, in Schizophrenia: Scientific Progress. Edited by Schultz SC, Tamminga CT. New York, Oxford University Press, 1989, pp 13–22

Carpenter WT Jr, Heinrichs DW, Wagman AMI: Deficit and nondeficit forms of schizophrenia: the concept. Am J Psychiatry 145:578–583, 1988

Chouinard G, Ross-Chouinard A, Annable L, et al: Extrapyramidal Symptom Rating Scale. Can J Neurol Sci 7:233, 1980

Chouinard G, Jones B, Remington G, et al: A Canadian multicenter placebo-controlled study of fixed doses of risperidone and haloperidol in the treatment of chronic schizophrenic patients. J Clin Psychopharmacol 13:25–40, 1993

Chiles JA, Miller AL, Crisom ML, et al: Development and implementation of the schizophrenia algorithm. Psychiatr Serv 50:69–74, 1999

Crow TJ: Molecular pathology of schizophrenia: more than one disease process? BMJ 280:66–68, 1980

Crow TJ: The two-syndrome concept: origins and current status. Schizophr Bull 11:471–486, 1985

De Hert M, Abrahams F, Fransen L, et al: Psychosis evaluation tool for common use by caregivers (PECC): development and validation. Schizophr Res 36:6, 1999

Spitzer RL, Endicott J: Schedule for Affective Disorders and Schizophrenia—Change Version (SADS-C), 3rd Edition. New York, Biometric Research, New York State Psychiatric Institute, 1978

Fenton WS, McGlashan TH: Testing systems for assessment of negative symptoms in schizophrenia. Arch Gen Psychiatry 49:179–184, 1992

Heresco-Levy U, Javitt DC, Ermilov M, et al: Double-blind, placebo-controlled, crossover trial of glycine adjuvant therapy for treatment-resistant schizophrenia. Br J Psychiatry 169:610–617, 1996

Iager A, Kirch DC, Wyatt RJ: A negative symptom rating scale. Psychiatry Res 16:27–36, 1985

Johnstone EC, Crow TJ, Frith CD, et al: The dementia of dementia praecox. Acta Psychiatr Scand 57:305–324, 1978

Kay SR, Opler LA, Fiszbein A: Significance of positive and negative syndromes in chronic schizophrenia. Br J Psychiatry 149:439–448, 1986

Kay SR, Fiszbein A, Opler LA: The Positive and Negative Syndrome Scale (PANSS) for schizophrenia. Schizophr Bull 13:261–276, 1987

Kirkpatrick B, Buchanan RW, McKenny PD, et al: The Schedule for the Deficit Syndrome: an instrument for research in schizophrenia. Psychiatry Res 30:119–123, 1989

Kirkpatrick B, Buchanan RW, Breier A, et al: Case identification and stability of the deficit syndrome of schizophrenia. Psychiatry Res 47:47–56, 1992

Knight RA, Roff JD: Affectivity in schizophrenia, in: Controversies in Schizophrenia. Edited by Alpert M. New York, Guilford, 1985

Kraepelin E: Dementia Praecox and Paraphrenia (1919). Translated by Barclay RM. Huntington, NY, RE Krieger, 1971

Krawiecka M, Goldberg D, Vaughan H: A standardized psychiatric assessment for rating chronic psychiatric patients. Acta Psychiatr Scand 55:299–308, 1977

Lewine RR, Fogg L, Meltzer HY: Assessment of negative and positive symptoms in schizophrenia. Schizophr Bull 9:368–378, 1983

Lindenmayer JP: Recent advances in pharmacotherapy of schizophrenia. Psychiatric Annals 23:201–208, 1993

Lindenmayer JP: The Positive and Negative Syndrome Scale: its use in psychopharmacological research. International Journal of Methods in Psychiatric Research 5:41–49, 1997

Lindenmayer JP, Kay SR: Depression, affective impairment, and negative symptoms in schizophrenia. Br J Psychiatry 155 (suppl 7):108–114, 1989

Lindenmayer JP, Bernstein-Hyman R, Grochowski S: Psychopathology of Schizophrenia: initial validation of a 5-factor model. Psychopathology 28:22–31, 1995

Marder SR, Meibach RC: Risperidone in the treatment of schizophrenia. Am J Psychiatry 151:825–835, 1994

Meltzer HY, Bastani B, Kwon KY, et al: A prospective study of clozapine in treatment-resistant schizophrenic patients, I: preliminary report. Psychopharmacology (Berl) 99 (suppl):S68–S72, 1989

Meltzer HY, Alphs LD, Bastani B, et al: Clinical efficacy of clozapine in the treatment of schizophrenia. Pharmacopsychiatry 24:44–45, 1991

Miller DD, Perry PJ, Cadoret RJ, et al: Clozapine's effect on negative symptoms in treatment-refractory schizophrenics. Compr Psychiatry 35:8–15, 1994

Möller H-J, Muller H, Borison RL, et al: A path-analytical approach to differentiate between direct and indirect drug effects on negative symptoms in schizophrenic patients: a re-evaluation of the North American risperidone study. Eur Arch Psychiatry Clin Neurosci 245:45–49, 1995

Nunnally JC: Psychometric Theory, 2nd Edition. New York, McGraw-Hill, 1978

Rak IW, Arvanitis LA: Overview of the efficacy of Seroquel (quetiapine). Schizophr Res 24:199, 1997

Tollefson GD, Beasley CM, Tran PV, et al: Olanzapine versus haloperidol: results of the multi-center international trial (abstract). Schizophr Res 18:131, 1996

Zimbroff DL, Kane JM, Tamminga CA, et al: Controlled, dose-response study of sertindole and haloperidol in the treatment of schizophrenia. Am J Psychiatry 154:782–791, 1997

Negative Symptoms and the Assessment of Neurocognitive Treatment Response

Richard S. E. Keefe, Ph.D.

Mr. G is a 34-year-old man with chronic schizophrenia. He developed symptoms of schizophrenia when he was 23. He had been employed as a short-order cook from ages 21–29, working at several different restaurants for a few months at a time before either being fired or quitting because of the anxiety he experienced while working during the busy times of the day. He eventually learned to request the "graveyard" shift, which was less busy. But even that work became too stressful for him. He found that he often forgot orders, and he sometimes would even forget what he was making while he was in the middle of cooking it. His worst problem was that when he had several orders to cook at once, he had great difficulty in developing a plan to organize all the orders at the same time. Sometimes he tried to cook too many dishes and would burn food. Other times he cooked too few orders, and angry customers would complain about him. The managers of the restaurants in which he worked usually became fed up with what they thought was his lazy attitude. Even those who knew he had a mental illness thought that he did not care about his work because he moved so much more slowly than the other cooks. When Mr. G tried to explain that he was moving as fast as he could, the managers did not believe him. Finally, Mr. G gave up on the idea that he could work. He has been unemployed for the past 5 years.

Like many patients with schizophrenia, Mr. G has significant cognitive deficits. Results of a neuropsychological testing battery suggest that his attention and verbal memory are very poor, with scores in the bottom 10%–15% range compared with people his age in the general population. Mr. G's working memory—that is, his ability to keep information in mind over brief periods of time—is also poor, with scores in the bottom 25% compared with normal). His ability to categorize information, make decisions, and construct plans is likewise poor, with scores in the bottom 10% compared with the general population. Anyone involved in Mr. G's treatment would be very concerned about his cognitive deficits and would be faced with the following questions: How much do these cognitive deficits affect Mr. G's life? Are they a result of his other symptoms of schizophrenia, such as his negative symptoms, or are they independent, warranting a treatment regimen specifically aimed at ameliorating them? Are medications available to treat these cognitive deficits? Will the improvements caused by these medications be clinically meaningful? What changes can Mr. G and his physician expect? How can the physician determine whether Mr. G's cognitive deficits are improving under his current treatment regimen?

This chapter is intended to benefit clinicians who face these types of questions during treatment or assessment of patients with schizophrenia and other psychotic disorders. The purpose of this chapter is to address the following three issues:

1. Are atypical antipsychotic medications superior to typical antipsychotics in their ability to improve cognitive dysfunction in schizophrenia? The results of a recently completed meta-analysis addressing this question will be described and discussed.
2. How is the degree of cognitive improvement produced by atypical antipsychotic medication clinically relevant, especially with regard to negative symptoms? The literature addressing this issue will be examined.
3. How can clinicians determine whether their patients are demonstrating cognitive improvement during a trial with a novel antipsychotic? A series of guidelines for assessing cognitive treatment response will be presented.

Question 1. Are atypical antipsychotics superior to typical antipsychotics in their ability to improve cognitive dysfunction in schizophrenia?

To address this first question empirically, a meta-analysis was conducted of the 15 studies that, as of June 30, 1998, had investigated the impact of novel antipsychotic medication on cognitive dysfunction in patients with schizophrenia (Keefe et al. 1999). The methodology and results of these studies are listed in Table 5–1. The analysis was not restricted to studies investigating a particular atypical antipsychotic medication. Three of the studies were randomized and double-blind, and 11 were open-label studies. In 1 study (Serper and Chou 1997) the patients on atypical antipsychotics, and a portion of the patients on haloperidol, were assessed in a double-blind manner; however, several of the patients on haloperidol were not so assessed. One of the open-label studies (Lee et al. 1994) used multiple study arms with random assignment. The numbers of studies examining each of the various atypical antipsychotics were as follows: clozapine, 11 studies; risperidone, 4 studies; zotepine, 1 study; ziprasidone, 1 study; and aripiprazole, 1 study. At the time this meta-analysis was conducted, published data from studies of olanzapine and quetiapine were not yet available.

A wide range of test measures was used in the 15 studies. Some studies employed only a few neurocognitive measures, while others conducted a more comprehensive neuropsychological assessment. The number of different neurocognitive tests included in a study ranged from 1 to 13.

Because of the variability in the type and number of measures used to assess neurocognitive effects, test results were grouped into the following categories: 1) attention subprocesses, 2) executive function, 3) working memory, 4) learning and memory; 5) visuospatial analysis, 6) verbal fluency, 7) digit-symbol substitution, and 8) fine motor function.

Review of Study Results

Each study was examined to determine improvement in performance of a single test after treatment with atypical antipsychotic medication versus after treatment with conventional antipsychotic medication (atypical vs. conventional) or a significant positive change in performance after treatment with conventional antipsychotic medication relative to baseline (atypical treatment only). Our definition of improvement was conservative. We corrected for multiple comparisons in each study using an experiment-wise P value of $<.05$, even if this statistical procedure was not used by the study's authors. For example, if 10 measures were reported in a study, we assigned a significance criterion of $.05/10 = .005$ for each measure.

The number of studies that assessed each neurocognitive domain is listed in Table 5–2, along with the number of studies that demonstrated significant improvements overall and in each of the cognitive domains. After we corrected for multiple comparisons, 9 of the 15 studies demonstrated significant neu-

TABLE 5–1. Characteristics and results of 15 studies of the effect of atypical antipsychotic medication on cognitive functions in patients with schizophrenia

Studies	Diagnosis of subjects	Baseline neurocognitive assessment (medication status)	Multiple study arms with random assignment	Double-blind condition	Trial duration	Medication and daily dose	Sample size	Reported neurocognitive improvements	Neurocognitive improvements after correction for multiple comparisons
Double blind (N=3)									
Meyer-Lindenberg et al. 1997	Treatment-resistant schizophrenia	Yes (4-day washout)	Yes	Yes	Testing at day 2, then weekly for 6 weeks	Clozapine 150–450 mg; zotepine 150–450 mg	26	Executive and fine motor	None
Buchanan et al. 1994 (phase I)	Treatment-responsive schizophrenia	Yes (fluphenazine)	Yes	Yes	10 weeks	Clozapine 400 mg (200–600 mg); haloperidol 20 mg (10–30 mg)	19 subjects in each group	Verbal fluency and visuospatial analysis (corrections for multiple comparisons made in original report)	Verbal fluency and visuospatial analysis

TABLE 5–1. Characteristics and results of 15 studies of the effect of atypical antipsychotic medication on cognitive functions in patients with schizophrenia (*continued*)

Studies	Diagnosis of subjects	Baseline neurocognitive assessment (medication status)	Multiple study arms with random assignment	Double-blind condition	Trial duration	Medication and daily dose	Sample size	Reported neurocognitive improvements	Neurocognitive improvements after correction for multiple comparisons
Green et al. 1997; McGurk et al. 1997; Kern et al. 1998	Treatment-resistant schizophrenia	Yes (3- to 7-day washout following 3-week haloperidol stabilization)	Yes	Yes	4 weeks	Risperidone 6 mg; haloperidol 15 mg	59	Attention, executive, motor functions	Attention
Open label (*N* = 12)									
Goldberg et al. 1993	Psychotic disorders	Yes (conventional antipsychotics)	No	No	3–24 months (mean 15 months)	Clozapine; many adjunctive medications	15	None	None
Hagger et al. 1993	Treatment-resistant schizophrenia	Yes (27 drug free; 5 conventional antipsychotics; 4 clozapine for 1–3 days)	No	No	6 weeks; 6 months; 1 year	Clozapine 363 mg ± 211 mg for 6 weeks; 403 mg ± 208 mg for 6 months	36	Executive function, attention, verbal fluency, and digit symbol	Verbal fluency; digit symbol

TABLE 5–1. Characteristics and results of 15 studies of the effect of atypical antipsychotic medication on cognitive functions in patients with schizophrenia (*continued*)

Studies	Diagnosis of subjects	Baseline neurocognitive assessment (medication status)	Multiple study arms with random assignment	Double-blind condition	Trial duration	Medication and daily dose	Sample size	Reported neurocognitive improvements	Neurocognitive improvements after correction for multiple comparisons
Buchanan et al. 1994 (phase II)	Treatment-responsive schizophrenia	Yes (fluphenazine)	No	No	1 year	Clozapine 200–600 mg	33	Visuospatial analysis, executive function, and verbal fluency	Verbal fluency
Lee et al. 1994	Treatment-responsive schizophrenia	Yes	Yes	No	6 weeks; 6 months; 1 year	Not available	Conventional: (n = 23); clozapine: (n = 24)	Executive, learning/memory, verbal fluency, and digit symbol	Executive, verbal fluency, digit symbol
Zahn et al. 1994	Schizophrenia	Yes (fluphenazine or placebo)	No	No	6 weeks each phase	Fluphenazine: mean 23 mg ± 14.8 mg; clozapine: mean 444 mg ± 189 mg	25	Attention	None

TABLE 5-1. Characteristics and results of 15 studies of the effect of atypical antipsychotic medication on cognitive functions in patients with schizophrenia (*continued*)

Studies	Diagnosis of subjects	Baseline neuro-cognitive assessment (medication status)	Multiple study arms with random assignment	Double-blind condition	Trial duration	Medication and daily dose	Sample size	Reported neuro-cognitive improvements	Neurocognitive improvements after correction for multiple comparisons
Gallhofer et al. 1996	Schizophrenia	No	No	No	7 days	Clozapine 200–400 mg; risperidone 4–8 mg; haloperidol 3–15 mg; fluphenazine 6–24 mg	16	Executive and fine motor	Executive and fine motor
Hoff et al. 1996	Treatment-resistant schizophrenia	Yes (conventional antipsychotics)	No	No	12 weeks	Baseline CPZ equivalents: 1,418 mg ± 809 mg; clozapine 425–900 mg (mean 668 mg ± 164 mg)	20	Verbal fluency and digit symbol	None

TABLE 5–1. Characteristics and results of 15 studies of the effect of atypical antipsychotic medication on cognitive functions in patients with schizophrenia *(continued)*

Studies	Diagnosis of subjects	Baseline neurocognitive assessment (medication status)	Multiple study arms with random assignment	Double-blind condition	Trial duration	Medication and daily dose	Sample size	Reported neurocognitive improvements	Neurocognitive improvements after correction for multiple comparisons
Stip and Lussier 1996	Schizophrenia	Yes (conventional antipsychotics)	No	No	8 weeks; 20–30 weeks	Haloperidol: variable dosages; 1 patient 40 mg; risperidone: variable dosages; 1 patient 11 mg, 2 patients 10 mg	13	Attention	Attention
Rossi et al. 1997	Schizophrenia	Yes (1 week placebo)	No	No	4 weeks	Risperidone 2 mg	$N = 30$	Executive, working memory, and digit symbol	Digit symbol
Serper and Chou 1997	Schizophrenia	Yes (medication free; time period unknown)	No	No	4 weeks	CPZ equivalents: 827 mg ± 528 mg; ziprasidone NA; aripiprazole NA	Atypical: ($n = 9$); conventional: ($n = 12$)	Attention	None

TABLE 5–1. Characteristics and results of 15 studies of the effect of atypical antipsychotic medication on cognitive functions in patients with schizophrenia *(continued)*

Studies	Diagnosis of subjects	Baseline neuro-cognitive assessment (medication status)	Multiple study arms with ran-dom as-signment	Double-blind condition	Trial duration	Medication and daily dose	Sample size	Reported neuro-cognitive im-provements	Neurocogni-tive improve-ments after correction for multiple comparisons
Galletly et al. 1997	Schizo-phrenia	Yes (1 medica-tion-free; 4 risperi-done; 14 convention-al antipsy-chotics)	No	No	6.5 months ± 2.0 months	Clozapine mean 393 mg ± 182 mg	19	Digit symbol, visuospatial processing, abstraction, verbal fluency, verbal work-ing memory, verbal delayed recall	None
Fujii et al. 1997	Treatment-resistant schizo-phrenia	Yes (conven-tional anti-psychotics)	No	No	12–16 months	Clozapine 250–900 mg (mean 643 mg)	10	Abstraction, digit symbol, intelligence (estimated total, verbal, and perfor-mance IQ)	Total IQ

Note. CPZ = chlorpromazine.

TABLE 5–2.   Study results by neurocognitive domain

Neurocognitive domains	Total number of studies	Number of studies reporting clinical improvement	Number of studies demonstrating improvement after correction for multiple comparisons
Any neurocognitive domain	15	14	9
Attention subprocesses	6	4	2
Executive function	12	8	2
Learning and memory	9	3	0
Working memory	3	2	0
Visuospatial analysis	5	3	1
Verbal fluency	6	6	4
Digit-symbol substitution	7	6	3
Fine motor function	3	2	1
Intelligence/IQ	4	1	1

rocognitive improvement on at least one test measure in response to atypical antipsychotic medication versus conventional antipsychotic treatment.

Meta-Analysis

The meta-analytic procedures used to examine the results of these studies statistically are described in detail in Keefe et al. (1999). Briefly, the Fisher method for combining *P* values was used; it provides a summary of the statistical significance of the results and a test of the null hypothesis that there is no difference between the effects of atypical antipsychotics and those of conventional antipsychotics. When a given study included multiple test measures, the average *P* value for that study was used in the statistical procedure. If multiple test measures were included in a single domain of cognitive functioning, the average *P* value for that domain was used in the statistical procedure. When *P* values were not available, we calculated them using the published means and standard deviations. In one case, we contacted the authors to obtain unpublished means and standard deviations.

The meta-analysis of the 15 studies indicated that atypical antipsychotics were significantly more effective than conventional antipsychotics in their ability to improve cognitive functioning (chi-square $= 62.41$, $P = .0004$). The effect of novel antipsychotics on specific domains of cognitive function was also examined by combining all studies that reported data for each domain. Corrections for multiple comparisons were not made, since doing so would have required setting a variable P value for each domain. Meta-analyses indicated significant improvements in attention, executive functions, working memory, visuospatial analysis, verbal fluency, digit-symbol substitution, fine motor functions, and visuospatial analysis with atypical antipsychotics (Keefe et al. 1999).

Conclusions From Review of Studies and Meta-Analysis

Despite our use of the very conservative statistical approach of correcting the results of each study for the number of statistical comparisons made, this meta-analysis strongly suggests that unlike conventional antipsychotics, atypical antipsychotics improve cognitive functions in patients with schizophrenia. The measures showing the strongest response to novel antipsychotics were verbal fluency, digit-symbol substitution, fine motor functions, and executive functions. Attention subprocesses were also responsive. Learning and memory functions were the least responsive.

The pattern of responsiveness of these functions suggests that measures with a timed component may be particularly responsive to novel antipsychotics. This pattern may be a result of the absence of extrapyramidal side effects (EPS) with atypical antipsychotic medications compared with conventional antipsychotics—that is, because all timed tests involve some degree of dependence on motor skills, which are impaired by EPS, the improved performance could partially be explained by the reduced EPS with atypical antipsychotics. Furthermore, the advantage of atypical antipsychotics over conventional antipsychotics may also be related to the absence of practice-related improvements in patients taking conventional antipsychotics. Although conventional antipsychotics may cause mild worsening of some aspects of cognitive function in patients with schizophrenia (Levin et al. 1996), they do not have direct and severe deleterious effects on cognition (Cassens et al. 1990; Medalia et al. 1988). However, conventional antipsychotics may be inferior to atypical antipsychotics in that they impair motor skills and prevent adequate learning effects.

Because of the limited number of studies included in our analysis, it is difficult to determine conclusively the pattern of specific cognitive improvements that can be expected with any specific atypical antipsychotic. However, there is preliminary support for the notion that clozapine is especially effective in improving motor skills and verbal fluency, and that risperidone may have particularly strong effects on attention and executive functions. As reported by Purdon et al. (2000) and reviewed in Meltzer and McGurk (1999), preliminary data suggest that olanzapine may also have beneficial cognitive effects.

The findings of this meta-analysis should be placed in the context of the fact that none of the 15 studies met all of the recently developed standards for the assessment of cognitive change in schizophrenia. Most importantly, only 3 of the 15 studies used double-blind methodology. The impact of the various rater biases inherent to open-label studies of patients with schizophrenia, underscored recently in the Department of Veterans Affairs collaborative study of clozapine (Rosenheck et al. 1997), may be strong. Nonetheless, these 15 studies have served a very important function. They have lent support to the relatively recent notion that cognitive impairment can be improved in patients with schizophrenia. As a result of these initial studies, several large-scale, comprehensive investigations of the effect of atypical antipsychotics on cognitive impairment in schizophrenia are currently under way. The results of these studies will be of great interest.

Question 2. How is the degree of cognitive improvement from atypical antipsychotic medication clinically relevant, especially with regard to negative symptoms?

Mr. G, the schizophrenia patient introduced at the beginning of this chapter, had suffered from severe cognitive deficits for 14 years. These cognitive deficits were relatively stable over time. In contrast, his hallucinations and delusions became quite severe during periods of psychotic exacerbation but remitted completely at times. Surprisingly, however, his social life and work life were relatively unaffected by the fluctuations of his psychosis. At times, he could work quite well while hallucinating. The worsening of his social and work functioning were caused by his persistent inability to pay attention, remember what he had learned, and organize the information that he did obtain. Over time, he became completely uninterested in working and socializing and even lost his ability to enjoy recreational activities. He became reclusive and had trouble taking care of his basic needs by himself. He was fortunate to have an older sister who had always looked after him. Otherwise, he very likely would have joined the millions of other patients with schizophrenia living on the streets.

The relationship between cognitive dysfunction and negative symptoms is complex, and there is a great deal about this relationship that is not understood. It has been well established, however, that various types of negative symptoms are strongly correlated with cognitive dysfunction (Addington et al. 1991; Braff et al. 1991; Manschreck et al. 1985; Cuesta and Peralta 1995; Strauss 1993; Morris et al. 1995). Global and specific aspects of cognitive dysfunction are significantly more likely to be correlated with negative symptoms than with positive symptoms (Addington et al. 1991; Braff et al. 1991; Tamlyn et al. 1992). As described by Trumbetta and Mueser (see Chapter 3 in this volume), a variety of reports have focused on the strong relationship between cognitive function and social deficits in schizophrenia. Patients with cognitive disturbances are certainly more likely than those without such dysfunction to have difficulties with interpersonal relationships and social situations.

The relationship between amotivation and cognitive deficits in schizophrenia is controversial. One point of contention is whether the negative symptom of amotivation underlies schizophrenia patients' poor performance on cognitive tests. In other words, do these patients perform poorly because they are less motivated to perform well on the tests they are given? The answer to this question appears to be mostly no. Monetary reinforcement has been found to improve the performance of schizophrenic patients on effortful cognitive measures such as the Wisconsin Card Sorting Test (WCST; Heaton 1981) in some studies (Summerfelt et al. 1991) but not in others (Green et al. 1990; Bellack et al. 1990). On tests that are less difficult, the performance of schizophrenic patients appears not to be affected by motivation (Schwartz et al. 1990; Tamlyn et al. 1992).

An index of pupillary response has been used as an indication of whether an individual is able to process information adequately (Granholm et al. 1996). Increases in pupil size are associated with increased cognitive-processing demands; pupil size begins to decline when the demands of the task exceed the processing resources available. Thus, pupillary responses can be used to determine whether an individual is sufficiently engaged in a task to perform adequately. If the cognitive deficits of schizophrenic patients were due to lack of interest or motivation, we would expect that their pupillary responses would be low throughout the period of cognitive assessment. However, patients with schizophrenia demonstrate normal pupillary responses during the low-processing conditions of a working memory task (Granholm et al. 1996). It is only during high-processing conditions that these patients show abnormal pupillary responses. These results suggest that although schizophrenic patients put forth a normal amount of effort during cognitive tests, their decreased processing capacity renders them unable to engage in difficult tasks.

The cognitive deficits of schizophrenia do not appear to be accounted for by reduced motivation. Rather, it seems likely that the causal relation between these two factors is in the opposite direction. Schizophrenia patients with cognitive deficits may be less motivated to set goals and pursue them. Those patients with severe cognitive deficits are likely to meet with failure if they attempt to pursue employment, social, and even recreational avenues that require cognitive skill. Such repeated failure would cause discouragement and reduced motivation even in people without mental illness.

If indeed cognitive deficits underlie amotivation, it is likely that treatment of cognitive deficits with atypical antipsychotic medication will increase these patients' motivation. Because cognitive deficits appear to continue to improve over the course of months of treatment (Buchanan et al. 1994), it would be unreasonable to expect motivation to improve dramatically during a brief trial of atypical antipsychotic treatment. It would be more beneficial to allow ample time for patients' cognitive deficits to improve, thus permitting subsequent improvements in motivation (Kane et al. 1988; Lieberman et al. 1994).

Impaired motor functions are a very important component of the profile of cognitive deficits in patients with schizophrenia. Motor slowing not only has social consequences for patients but also can dramatically affect their ability to perform basic work tasks adequately. Like Mr. G, the patient in our example, many patients with schizophrenia are both embarrassed about their motor impairments and severely disabled by them. Empirical studies suggest that motor functions are strongly correlated with negative symptoms (Manschreck et al. 1985; Morris et al. 1995) and with outcome (Bilder et al. 1985). To some extent, deficient motor skills are represented in both the negative symptom and the cognitive dysfunction domain, given that symptoms such as blunted affect and motor retardation are actually observational measures of motor functioning. Thus, impaired motor skills in many ways lie at the core of negative symptoms in schizophrenia.

It should be noted that the relationship between motor skills deficits and negative symptoms may be partially explained by EPS. The association between greater severity of negative symptoms and poorer performance on motor tasks is stronger for patients on typical antipsychotics than for patients who have had their medications withdrawn (Himmelhoch et al. 1996).

In sum, cognitive deficits and negative symptoms are correlated in a broad variety of areas. The important question regards the way in which improvements in these two domains are related to one another. If a patient demonstrates improvement in cognitive abilities, what kind of improvement can be expected in negative symptoms and functioning?

Following a 6-week trial with an atypical antipsychotic medication, Mr. G began to show signs of improved cognitive functioning. He started to remember phone numbers, which had previously been impossible for him. He was now able to watch a half-hour television show in its entirety, whereas before, he had frequently stopped paying attention, lost interest, and then bothered his family members by talking during the important parts of the show. After 6 months on the new medication, Mr. G began to feel a spark of life that had been missing for a long time. He felt more alert and interested in sporting events again. He seemed to move more quickly; a neighbor noted that Mr. G no longer seemed to shuffle around like he used to, and his sister noted that he seemed to have "a bounce in his step." He came home one night very proud that he had been able to give directions to a woman who had become lost driving in her car. Mr. G began to move and think with enough competence that he started cooking dinner regularly for his sister's family. One morning, his sister found him looking in the classified section of the paper. He said he was "just curious" whether there were any short-order-cook jobs in the area.

If atypical antipsychotic medication indeed improves cognition, the benefit is not limited to performance on psychological tests. Cognitive improvement betters patients' lives. It would seem to make sense that if atypical antipsychotic treatment improves patients' ability to pay attention, remember, and understand the world around them, their interest in the outside world and their ability to function in it will naturally improve. This association was demonstrated empirically in a 1-year clozapine study conducted by Buchanan and colleagues (1994). In that study, a significant relationship was found between improvement in verbal memory and improvement in Quality of Life Scale (QLS; Heinrichs et al. 1984) scores following a full year of treatment with clozapine. Patients whose memories improved tended to report a better quality of life; patients whose memories worsened tended to report a worsened quality of life. It is unlikely—though not impossible—that improvements in quality of life caused memory enhancement in these patients. A more probable explanation is that memory improvement over the course of a year allowed patients to improve the quality of their lives.

An association between cognitive improvement and negative symptom reduction with atypical antipsychotic medication was reported in three of the six studies that investigated this relationship statistically. Negative symptom reduction was associated with improvements in verbal fluency and digit-symbol substitution in two separate studies (Galletly et al. 1997; Hagger et al. 1993) and with improvements in verbal memory and executive functions in one study (Hagger et al. 1993). Improvements in anergia and motor speed were also found to be associated with negative symptom improvement in a third study (Gallhofer et al. 1996). It is interesting to note that several of the cognitive tests used in these studies have a timed component, which suggests that the relationship between negative symptom improvement and cognitive improvement may be attributable to the impact of atypical antipsychotic medication on motor speed.

Question 3. How can clinicians determine whether their patients are demonstrating cognitive improvement during a trial with a novel antipsychotic?

Although no specific battery of cognitive tests designed to measure the degree of cognitive improvement with atypical antipsychotics is currently available, studies are under way to develop such a battery, and it should be available in the near future. The question often arises, however, of how clinical psychiatrists can determine whether their patients have demonstrated the level of cognitive enhancement that can be expected with atypical antipsychotic medication. The remainder of this chapter will address this question.

Pharmacological Status at Baseline

A clinical assessment of the impact of atypical antipsychotics on cognitive function must consider patients' treatment status prior to the initiation of the new medication. Because conventional antipsychotics have repeatedly been found to be only minimally effective in improving cognitive function (Cassens et al. 1990; Medalia et al. 1988) and may even worsen some aspects of cognition (Levin et al. 1996), any improvements observed can be attributed to the atypical agent. Whereas in individuals without schizophrenia, repeated administrations of some cognitive tests can lead to better scores, schizophrenia patients on typical antipsychotics rarely show these practice effects. Thus, for most tests, improvements with atypical antipsychotics will not be attributable to simple practice effects. During baseline assessment, it is acceptable to allow patients to remain on their usual adjunctive medications. If treatment with a specific agent increases the likelihood that patients will receive a particular form of adjunctive medication that has a cognitive effect, then the emergence of this cognitive effect can be viewed as being indirectly caused by that agent. For example, if treatment with conventional antipsychotics increases the likelihood that patients will require anticholinergic medication, which impairs memory (McEvoy et al. 1987; Strauss et al. 1990), then those memory impairments can be fairly attributed to the conventional antipsychotic treatment. However, patients should not be evaluated while on adjunctive medications that are rarely administered to them. Doing so could misrepresent the actual profile of the patient's cognitive deficits. For example, one-time administration of benzodiazepines to alleviate anxiety during cognitive testing is not suggested, since the resultant cognitive state is not representative of the patient's usual cognitive state while on the antipsychotic medication of interest.

The baseline assessment should be conducted after a period of stability in the patients' medication regimen. Patients who have recently undergone a change in medication or dosage are more likely to experience uncontrolled side effects and acute symptom exacerbation. Thus, it is not ideal to assess the cognitive functions of acutely admitted patients who have been on their current treatment regimen for only a few days. Harvey and Keefe (P. D. Harvey and R. S. E. Keefe, "Studies of Cognitive Change With Novel Antipsychotic Treatment in Schizophrenia" [unpublished paper], June 2000) recommend a 4- to 6-week period of stable treatment before conducting a baseline assessment. The exception to this standard is the assessment of patients who have not taken their medication for an unspecified period of time. In this case, it is important to determine baseline levels of clinical symptoms to assess the relationship between a patient's improvement in baseline psychopathology and cognitive improvement.

Choice of Medication

The choice of which atypical antipsychotic should be used in a given patient is complex. At present, although it is certain that atypical antipsychotics improve cognitive functioning, there is no clear favorite among those currently available. The review of the literature presented above suggested that risperidone may have an advantage in executive functions and attention, whereas clozapine may have an advantage in functions involving motor abilities. Olanzapine may also have advantages in tests of attention and tests with a speed or motor component. Notwithstanding these hints, if there are great differences among the atypical antipsychotics in their ability to enhance cognition, these have not yet been brought to light. In the coming years, several large-sample studies will be completed, and these will provide a clearer profile of each medication's strengths and weaknesses in improving cognition. At some point, it may even be possible to prescribe specific medications based on the convergence of a patient's areas of cognitive dysfunction and a medication's ability to improve those specific areas of dysfunction.

Objective Evaluation

One of the great advantages of using psychological tests to measure improvements in cognition is that the tests are objective. Thus, they are far superior to clinical impressions that a patient's cognitive function has improved, given that such impressions can be based on factors unrelated to cognition. This bias may be particularly evident when a patient and a clinician are so eager for improvements to occur that they believe they see them even when there has been no change. However, psychological tests are useful only if they are administered properly. Most psychologists with clinical training have the necessary expertise to administer psychological tests. In some cases, technicians can administer tests with extensive supervision from a psychologist, but they also usually need input from a psychologist to interpret the test scores. Even the evaluation of cognitive functions with repeated administrations of the same tests can yield scores that require expert interpretation.

On the other hand, a disadvantage of most psychological tests is that inherent in each score is some degree of error. Thus, small improvements need to be viewed cautiously, because they may attributable to factors unrelated to the medication change. Such confounding factors include time of day the tests are administered, events in the patient's life that may affect his or her mood, subclinical changes in symptoms, recent alcohol or drug use, and many others. Finally, any improvements (or decrements) in performance need to be followed up with later testing. If a patient's cognitive functions have really improved, the change should remain stable or even be greater with subsequent testing.

Adequate Duration of Trial

The response of psychotic and negative symptoms has been reported to continue for months after the initiation of atypical antipsychotic treatment in some studies (Lieberman et al. 1994; Wilson 1996), but not others (Conley et al. 1997). It is possible that cognitive functions may also continue to improve over this time frame (Buchanan et al. 1994). For this reason, the assessment of the long-term impact of atypical antipsychotics on cognitive functions is very important. Furthermore, complex cognitive functions (e.g. executive functions) that depend on adequate cognitive skill in several areas may require longer periods of time to show improvement. Finally, it is possible that important outcome factors such as employment and independent living may improve only after long periods of enhanced cognitive function. Ideally, assessment should occur at 6 weeks, 12 weeks, 6 months, and 1 year following the initiation of atypical antipsychotic medication.

Clinically Appropriate Dosing Strategies

The comparison of two medications, one of which is appropriately dosed, and the other of which is inappropriately dosed, could provide potentially misleading results. For example, it is not informative to compare a patient's baseline performance on 40 mg/day of haloperidol with the patient's performance on a properly dosed atypical antipsychotic, because the high haloperidol dosage does not allow the patient to perform at an optimum level, particularly on tasks with a motor component. Likewise, although the manufacturer's initial suggested dose for risperidone was 6–16 mg/day, subsequent studies determined that patients often developed EPS at the higher end of this dose range, prompting a recommendation that the range be reduced to 0.5–6.0 mg/day. Studies of cognitive improvement with atypical antipsychotics must use the most recent information available regarding appropriate dosage ranges (Keefe et al. 1999).

Appropriate Neurocognitive Test Batteries

To be considered appropriate, a neurocognitive battery must 1) include measures that are among the many on which patients with schizophrenia show impairment, 2) have statistical and distributional properties that allow improvement with treatment, and 3) have a number of measures that is neither so small that important improvements will be easily missed nor so large that time and resources will be wasted on less-relevant tests.

Content

There are many potentially important areas of cognitive functioning in patients with schizophrenia. A good battery of tests will include tests that measure all of the domains listed in Table 5–3. Tests of vigilance, executive functions, and verbal memory may be particularly important because of their demonstrated relationship with aspects of outcome (Green 1996). It is also important to include measures that previous studies have suggested *should* be responsive to the medication of interest. For example, an assessment of the effectiveness of clozapine or risperidone should certainly include tests of verbal fluency and digit-symbol substitution, since schizophrenia patients undergoing trials with these medications have demonstrated improvements in these tests. If a patient is taking adjunctive medications that have specific cognitive

TABLE 5–3.   Guidelines for the clinical assessment of cognitive change in patients with schizophrenia

1. Pharmacological status at baseline assessment
    Treatment and symptom stability prior to assessment
    Conventional antipsychotic in most patients
    Allow chronically administered adjunctive medications
    Discontinue acutely administered or sporadically administered medications
      prior to assessment
2. Choice of medication
3. Objective evaluation
    Psychologist or trained technician to administer battery
    Psychologist interpretation of cognitive data
    Small changes treated with caution
    Assess the stability of the change with subsequent assessments
4. Adequate duration of trial
    Short-term and long-term assessments
5. Clinically appropriate dosing strategies
6. Appropriate neurocognitive test batteries

    A. Content
        Include measures that are expected to improve
        Include measures that correlate with functional outcome
        Include measures sensitive to potential adjunctive treatment
    B. Properties
        Available normative data
        Test–retest reliability
        Absence of ceiling or floor effects
        Brief presentation
    C. Number of tests
        Minimum number that can assess all relevant cognitive functions

7. Response criteria
    Expectations for response based on baseline cognitive deficits, age, and
      education
8. Discrimination between cognitive improvement and other clinical changes
    Negative symptoms
    Positive symptoms
    Medication side effects

effects, such as anticholinergic medication, it would be useful to include tests of memory in the assessment battery, since these functions would be expected to improve when atypical antipsychotics are initiated and anticholinergics are discontinued.

Properties

Tests used in a clinical assessment of the effect of atypical antipsychotic medications should have the following statistical and distributional properties:

available normative data, test–retest reliability, absence of ceiling or floor effects, and brief presentation. These properties will ensure that improvement (or absence of improvement) in patients' performance is attributable to the actual change (or absence of change) in their cognitive status. Tests with ceiling effects are particularly problematic. Patients who perform as well as possible on a test that is too easy will then have no room to improve. Thus, the medication recently administered to the patient will have no opportunity to enhance the cognitive function being measured.

Number of Tests

Finally, the number of outcome measures used can vary but should be large enough so that the impact of an atypical antipsychotic can be determined on a range of cognitive functions. On the other hand, the battery should be short enough so that psychotic patients can complete it without decrements in energy and motivation. The factor most likely to determine successful completion of a battery is rater expectation. Thus, it is fruitful to ensure that testers feel comfortable enough with the battery length that they expect to be able to complete it.

Response Criteria

Criteria for cognitive function response to atypical antipsychotic medication have not been determined. It is important to note that the degree of cognitive enhancement experienced by a patient depends on several factors besides the new medication, such as baseline level of cognitive deficits, age, education, and the response of other symptom domains to the medication. Compared with patients who do well at baseline, patients who perform very poorly are more likely to perform better at follow-up, even if they are relatively unaffected by the medication change. Random error variance (also known as "regression to the mean") will dictate that the patients who perform poorly have a better chance to improve their performance the next time. Regarding age and education, older, less-educated patients may not have as healthy a cognitive and neural structure as younger, more-educated patients. Therefore, smaller improvements may be viewed as clinically significant in these groups.

The data published to date suggest that the average patient with schizophrenia does not demonstrate large improvements with atypical neuroleptic treatment. Many functions will not improve at all. Functions that can be expected to improve will demonstrate changes that on average will range between 0.2 and 1.0 standard deviations. (These changes correspond to IQ improvements of 3 points and 15 points, respectively). Verbal fluency and digit-symbol tests have repeatedly been demonstrated to improve by about 0.5 standard deviations on average (Hagger et al. 1993; Hoff et al. 1996; Rossi et al. 1997). Given that patients with schizophrenia perform about 2.0 standard deviations below the mean on these tests, these improvements cannot be considered large. Thus, in clinical assessments of these patients, small improvements can be deemed significant.

Discrimination Between Cognitive Improvement and Other Clinical Changes

Cognitive impairment is not independent from other aspects of the clinical picture in patients with schizophrenia. As reviewed earlier, cognitive deficits are associated with various negative symptoms. However, cognitive deficits are also associated with movement disorders (Sorokin et al. 1988; Spohn et al. 1988) and medication side effects (Walker and Green 1982; Earle-Boyer et al. 1991). Therefore, the extent to which cognitive change overlaps with changes in other symptom and side-effect domains should be evaluated in each patient. An excellent strategy is to assess positive, negative, and disorganized symptoms, as well as side effects and movement disorders, at each assessment in which the cognitive battery is administered. Change scores in cognitive measures can then be examined to determine the extent to which they are explained by changes in other aspects of the illness.

Summary and Conclusions

Our statistical analysis of the results from 15 studies suggests that atypical antipsychotic medication improves many different aspects of cognitive functioning in patients with schizophrenia. These improvements appear to be related to negative symptoms. Contrary to the popular belief that improvements in negative symptoms cause improvements on cognitive tests, it is possible that the basis of this relation is that improvements in cognitive function cause subsequent improvements in negative symptoms. Previous research suggesting that cognitive dysfunction is strongly related to outcome underscores the importance of improving cognitive functions in patients with schizophrenia. These improvements better the quality of patients' lives. Finally, with regard to the assessment of cognitive function treatment response, several imperatives apply. It is essential that medication trials be controlled, objective, and of adequate duration. The tests chosen for such assessments must be appropriate in terms of their content, properties, and number, and it is preferable that they be administered by a psychologist or by a technician supervised by a psychologist.

References

Addington J, Addington D, Maticka-Tyndale E: Cognitive functioning and positive and negative symptoms in schizophrenia. Schizophr Res 4:123–134, 1991

Bellack AS, Mueser KT, Morrison RL: Remediation of cognitive deficits in schizophrenia: training on the Wisconsin Card Sorting Test. Paper presented at the annual American College of Neuropsychopharmacology Annual Meeting, Maui, Hawaii, December 1990

Bilder RM, Mukherjee S, Rieder RO, et al: Symptomatic and neuropsychological components of defect states. Schizophr Bull 11:409–419, 1985

Braff DL, Heaton R, Kuck J, et al: The generalized pattern of neuropsychological deficits in outpatients with chronic schizophrenia with heterogeneous Wisconsin Card Sorting Test results. Arch Gen Psychiatry 48:891–898, 1991

Buchanan RW, Holstein C, Brier A: The comparative efficacy and long-term effect of clozapine treatment on neuropsychological test performance. Biol Psychiatry 36:717–725, 1994

Cassens G, Inglis AK, Appelbaum PS, et al: Effects on neuropsychological function in chronic schizophrenic patients. Schizophr Bull 16:477–500, 1990

Conley RR, Carpenter WT Jr, Tamminga CA: Time to clozapine response in a standardized trial. Am J Psychiatry 154:1243–1247, 1997

Cuesta MJ, Peralta V: Cognitive disorders in the positive, negative and disorganization syndromes of schizophrenia. Psychiatry Res 58:227–235, 1995

Earle-Boyer EA, Serper MR, Davidson M, et al: Auditory and visual continuous performance tests in medicated and unmedicated schizophrenic patients: clinical and motoric correlates. Psychiatry Res 37:47–56, 1991

Fujii DEM, Ahmed I, Jokumsen M, et al: The effects of clozapine on cognitive functioning in treatment-resistant schizophrenic patients. J Neuropsychiatry Clin Neurosci 9:240–245, 1997

Galletly CA, Clark RC, McFarlane AC, et al: The relationship between changes in symptom ratings, neuropsychological test performance, and quality of life in schizophrenic patients treated with clozapine. Psychiatry Res 72:161–166, 1997

Gallhofer B, Bauer U, Lis S, et al: Cognitive dysfunction in schizophrenia: comparison of treatment with atypical antipsychotic agents and conventional neuroleptic drugs. European Neuropsychopharmacology 6 (suppl 2):13–20, 1996

Goldberg TE, Greenberg RD, Griffin SJ, et al: The effect of clozapine on cognition and psychiatric symptoms in patients with schizophrenia. Br J Psychiatry 162:43–48, 1993

Granholm E, Asarnow RF, Andrew J, et al: Pupillary responses index cognitive resource limitations. Psychophysiology 33:457–461, 1996

Granholm E, Morris, SK, Sarkin AJ: Pupillary response index overload of working memory resources in schizophrenia. J Abnorm Psychol 106:458–467, 1997

Green MF: What are the functional consequences of neurocognitive deficits in schizophrenia? Am J Psychiatry 153:321–330, 1996

Green MF, Ganxzell S, Satz P, et al: Teaching the Wisconsin Card Sorting Test to schizophrenic patients. Arch Gen Psychiatry 47:91–92, 1990

Green MF, Marshall BD Jr, Wirshing WC, et al: Does risperidone improve verbal working memory in treatment-resistant schizophrenia? Am J Psychiatry 154:799–804, 1997

Hagger C, Buckley P, Kenny JT, et al: Improvement in cognitive functions and psychiatric symptoms in treatment-refractory schizophrenic patients receiving clozapine. Biol Psychiatry 34:702–712, 1993

Heaton RK: The Wisconsin Card Sorting Test. Odessa, FL, Psychological Resources, 1981

Heinrichs DW, Hanlon TE, Carpenter WT Jr: The Quality of Life Scale: an instrument for rating the schizophrenic deficit syndrome. Schizophr Bull 10:388–398, 1984

Himmelhoch S, Taylor SF, Goldman RS, et al: Frontal lobe tasks, antipsychotic medications and schizophrenia syndromes. Biol Psychiatry 39:227–229, 1996

Hoff AL, Faustman WO, Wieneke M, et al: The effects of clozapine on symptom reduction, neurocognitive function, and clinical management in treatment-refractory state hospital schizophrenic inpatients. Neuropsychopharmacology 15:361–369, 1996

Kane J, Honifeld G, Singer J, et al: Clozapine for the treatment-resistant schizophrenic: a double-blind comparison with chlorpromazine. Arch Gen Psychiatry 45:789–796, 1988

Keefe RSE, Silva SG, Perkins DO, et al: The effects of atypical antipsychotic drugs on neurocognitive impairment in schizophrenia: a review and meta-analysis. Schizophr Bull 25:201–222, 1999

Kern RS, Green MF, Marshall BD Jr, et al: Risperidone vs. haloperidol on reaction time, manual dexterity, and motor learning in treatment-resistant schizophrenia patients. Biol Psychiatry. 44:726–732, 1998

Lee MA, Thompson PA, Meltzer HY: Effects of clozapine on cognitive function in schizophrenia. J Clin Psychiatry 55 (suppl B):82–87, 1994

Levin ED, Wilson W, Rose JE, et al: Nicotine-haloperidol interactions and cognitive performance in schizophrenics. Neuropsychopharmacology 15:429–436, 1996

Lieberman JA, Safferman AZ, Pollack S, et al: Clinical effects of clozapine in chronic schizophrenia: response to treatment and predictors of outcome. Am J Psychiatry 151:1744–1752, 1994

Manschreck TC, Maher BA, Waller NG, et al: Deficient motor synchrony in schizophrenic disorders: clinical correlates. Biol Psychiatry 20:990–1002, 1985

McEvoy JP, McCue M, Spring CM, et al: Effects of amantadine and trihexyphenidyl on memory in elderly normal volunteers. Am J Psychiatry 144:573–577, 1987

McGurk SR, Green MF, Wirshing WC, et al: The effects of risperidone vs. haloperidol on cognitive function in treatment-resistant schizophrenia: the Trail Making Test. CNS Spectrums 2:60–64, 1997

Medalia A, Gold JM, Merriam A: The effects of neuroleptics on neuropsychological test results of schizophrenics. Archives of Clinical Neuropsychology 3:249–271, 1988

Meltzer HY, McGurk SR: The effect of clozapine, risperidone, and olanzapine on cognitive function in schizophrenia. Schizophr Bull 25:233–255, 1999

Morris RG, Rushe T, Woodruffe PW, et al: Problem solving in schizophrenia: a specific deficit in planning ability. Schizophr Res 14:235–246, 1995

Meyer-Lindenberg A, Gruppe H, Bauer U, et al: Improvement of cognitive function in schizophrenic patients receiving clozapine or zotepine: results from a double-blind study. Pharmacopsychiatry 30:35–42, 1997

Rosenheck R, Cramer J, Xu W, et al: A comparison of clozapine and haloperidol in hospitalized patients with refractory schizophrenia: Department of Veterans Affairs Cooperative Study Group on Clozapine in Refractory Schizophrenia. N Engl J Med 337:809–815, 1997

Rossi A, Mancini F, Stratta P, et al: Risperidone, negative symptoms and cognitive deficit in schizophrenia: an open study. Acta Psychiatr Scand 95:40–43, 1997

Schwartz BD, Livingston JE, Sautter F, et al: Sustained attention by schizophrenics. New Trends in Experimental and Clinical Psychiatry 6:169–176, 1990

Serper, MR, Chou JCY: Novel neuroleptics improve attentional functioning in schizophrenic patients: ziprasidone and aripiprazole. CNS Spectrums 2:56–59, 1997

Sorokin JE, Giordani B, Mohs RC, et al: Memory impairment in schizophrenic patients with tardive dyskinesia. Biol Psychiatry 23:129–135, 1988

Spohn HE, Coyne L, Spray J: The effect of neuroleptics and tardive dyskinesia on smooth-pursuit eye movement in chronic schizophrenics. Arch Gen Psychiatry 45:833–840, 1988

Stip E, Lussier I: The effect of risperidone on cognition in patients with schizophrenia. Can J Psychiatry 41 (8 suppl 2):S35–S40, 1996

Strauss ME: Relations of symptoms to cognitive deficits in schizophrenia. Schizophr Bull 19:215–231, 1993

Strauss ME, Reynolds KS, Jayaram G, et al: Effects of anticholinergic medication on memory in schizophrenia. Schizophr Res 3:127–129, 1990

Summerfelt AT, Alphs LD, Funderburk FR, et al: Impaired Wisconsin Card Sort Performance in schizophrenia may reflect motivational deficits. Arch Gen Psychiatry 48:282–283, 1991

Tamlyn D, McKenna PJ, Mortimer AM, et al: Memory impairment in schizophrenia: its extent, affiliations, and neuropsychological character. Psychol Med 22:101–115, 1992

Walker E, Green MF: Motor proficiency and attention-task performance by schizophrenic patients. J Abnorm Psychol 91:261–268, 1982

Wilson WH: Time required for initial improvement during clozapine treatment of refractory schizophrenia. Am J Psychiatry 153:951–952, 1996

Zahn TP, Pickar D, Haier RJ: Effects of clozapine, fluphenazine, and placebo on reaction time measures of attention and sensory dominance in schizophrenia. Schizophr Res 13:133–144, 1994

6 Negative Symptoms and the Experience of Emotion

Christie Limpert, Ph.D.
Xavier F. Amador, Ph.D.

Negative symptoms are of tremendous clinical importance. Research suggests that negative symptoms are associated with poorer outcome (Fenton and McGlashan 1992, 1994; for reviews, see McGlashan and Fenton 1992 and Pogue-Geile and Zubin 1988) and that they may be less responsive to treatment with neuroleptic medication than are positive symptoms (Kane 1996; Kane and Freeman 1994; Kinon et al. 1993; Smith et al. 1996). Negative symptoms are also associated with a range of cognitive deficits (Bilder et al. 1985; Green and Walker 1985; Liddle 1987; Mayer et al. 1985) that may impair functioning in patients with schizophrenia. In an effort to refine the terminology of negative symptoms and provide a foundation for meaningful subtyping based on such symptoms, Carpenter et al. (1988) have divided negative symptoms into two categories: those thought to stem from the disorder itself (i.e., primary negative, or deficit symptoms) and those due to other, secondary causes, such as depression, neuromotor dysfunction, or medication side effects. As discussed throughout this volume, there are a number of different ways of conceptualizing negative symptoms. In this chapter, we argue that a diminished ability to experience emotion is a key characteristic of both negative and deficit symptomatology, with important implications for theory, assessment, and treatment. Impaired ability to experience emotion may be a domain of psychopathology that underlies other, more observable deficits, such as flat affect and social withdrawal; at the very least, diminished emotional experience is an added dimension of negative and deficit symptoms. Although relatively few studies have empirically exam-

111

ined the experience of emotion, we will present both research evidence and clinical material that suggests that diminished emotional experience is an important feature that characterizes at least a subgroup of patients with schizophrenia.

The experience of emotion is only one aspect of affective functioning. Although diminished emotional experience among patients with schizophrenia was considered important by early theorists, it has since been somewhat neglected and has not been the focus of much empirical work until recently. In the following sections, we review this literature and make an argument for the important methodological and clinical benefits of studying emotional experience in addition to other aspects of affective functioning in schizophrenia.

Historical Descriptions of Affective Deficits

Both Kraepelin (1919/1971) and Bleuler (1911/1950) conceptualized affective deficits as fundamental symptoms of schizophrenia, and both authors gave particular emphasis to diminished emotional experience. Kraepelin, for example, described emotional dullness in patients with dementia praecox, noting that

> the singular indifference of the patients towards their former emotional relations, the extinction of affection for relatives and friends, of satisfaction in their work and vocation, in recreation and pleasures, is not seldom the first and most striking symptom of the onset of disease. The patients have no real joy in life, "no human feelings"; to them "nothing matters, everything is the same"; they feel "no grief and no joy," "their heart is not in what they say." (Kraepelin 1919/1971, p. 33)

Similarly, Bleuler (1911/1950) noted that patients with schizophrenia often exhibited indifference toward relatives, friends, jobs, and pleasurable activities. These authors described diminished emotional experience as a primary symptom of schizophrenia—that is, as stemming directly from the disease itself. Bleuler's descriptions of patients emphasized the diminished ability to experience pleasure, whereas Kraepelin's descriptions highlighted the loss of both positive and negative emotional experiences. Later theorists also gave prominence to loss of positive emotional experiences, or anhedonia, conceptualizing it as a characterological deficit that reflected a genetic predisposition to the development of schizophrenia, rather than a symptom of the illness itself (Meehl 1962; Rado 1956). Meehl (1975), for example, argued that the ability to experience pleasure (hedonic capacity) is a trait that is normally distributed in the population and that those individuals at the lower extreme of the curve (i.e., those with diminished hedonic capacity) have a greater chance of developing schizophrenia.

Despite the seeming historical importance of diminished emotional experience in the characterization of schizophrenia, this deficit, as well as affective deficits in a more general sense, has been largely ignored by many contemporary diagnostic systems. Various classifications of the symptoms of schizophrenia have emphasized thought disorder over affective deficits (Feighner et al. 1972; K. Schneider 1959; Spitzer et al. 1977). It was only relatively recently, in the third revised edition of the *Diagnostic and Statistical Manual of Mental Disorders* (DSM-III-R; American Psychiatric Association 1987), that affective disturbances (i.e., flat or grossly inappropriate affect) were included as characteristic symptoms of the illness. In the most recent edition of the manual (DSM-IV; American Psychiatric Association 1994), the definition of characteristic symptoms has been broadened to include avolition and alogia in addition to flat affect. In previous editions, affective disturbance was considered only as a prodromal or residual symptom. In a parallel vein, research examining the nature of affective deficits in schizophrenia has become a focus of interest within the field only relatively recently. This neglect of affective deficits in research and practice seems to be related, at least in part, to the difficulty of operationalizing and measuring emotional constructs in a valid and reliable way. As we describe later in this chapter, improvements in the methodology for assessing such symptoms have resulted in numerous advances in our understanding of affective deficits in schizophrenia.

With the explosion of research and clinical interest in negative symptoms in recent years, there has also been renewed interest in affective deficits more generally. There is a general consensus that affective dysfunction is a fundamental aspect of negative symptoms, although theorists differ as to whether other, nonaffective symptoms should also be included under the heading of negative symptomatology (Malla 1995). In the following section, we review the literature on affective deficits in schizophrenia, with an emphasis on distinguishing deficits in emotional experience from deficits in other aspects of affective functioning.

Domains of Affective Deficit

Affective deficits can be divided into three general domains: 1) deficits in the *perception* of emotion (i.e., difficulty judging and interpreting the emotional displays of others), 2) deficits in the *expression* of emotion (i.e., difficulty conveying one's emotional experience to others), and 3) deficits in the *experience* of emotion (i.e., difficulty with the subjective feeling of emotion). A large body of research, which we review below, suggests that patients with schizophrenia exhibit deficits in all three of these domains. However, research in these areas has been conducted mostly independently, with few studies examining the interrelationships of the three domains. In addition, perhaps because of the difficulty inherent in measuring inner states, investigators have tended to neglect the experiential domain. Despite these difficulties, we will argue that the assessment of subjective emotional experience is a vital area for further empirical study. Moreover, we believe that such assessment has the potential to provide the clinician with valuable information for conceptualizing and treating patients with schizophrenia.

The Perception and Expression of Emotion

Deficits in Perception

The greatest amount of empirical work has been conducted in the area of perception of emotion. Despite using a variety of different methods, these studies have generally reported that schizophrenia patients demonstrate impairments in the ability to accurately identify the facial and vocal emotional expressions of others. For example, numerous studies have found that schizophrenia patients are impaired relative to nonpsychiatrically ill control subjects in judging various facial expressions depicted in photographs (Borod et al. 1993, 1989, 1990; Cutting 1981; Dougherty et al. 1974; Feinberg et al. 1986; Gaebel and Wölwer 1992; Heimberg et al. 1992; Kerr and Neale 1993; Kline et al. 1992; Lewis and Garver 1995; Mandal and Palchoudhury 1985, 1989; Muzekari and Bates 1977; Novic et al. 1984; Pilowsky and Bassett 1980; Walker et al. 1980, 1984; Whittaker et al. 1994; Zuroff and Colussy 1986). Studies using videotaped scenes of actors as the stimuli to be judged have reported similar results (Bellack et al. 1992; Cramer et al. 1989, 1992; Hellewell et al. 1994; Muzekari and Bates 1977). Several studies also provide evidence for a deficit in judging vocal expressions of emotion in schizophrenia patients compared with controls (Borod et al. 1989, 1990; Haskins et al. 1995; Kerr and Neale 1993; Murphy and Cutting 1990; Novic et al. 1984).

Thus, although a great deal of evidence suggests that schizophrenia patients and nonpsychiatrically ill individuals differ in their performance on tasks involving perception of emotion, not all of the studies providing this evidence have used adequate controls. In order to argue that such differences reflect an affective dysfunction in schizophrenia, rather than impaired attention or general cognitive dysfunction, it is necessary to use adequate control tasks. In research on the perception of facially expressed emotion, many studies have employed facial recognition memory tasks as controls. Although a few studies have found that schizophrenia patients' performance is comparable to that of nonpsychiatrically ill people on such tasks (Kline et al. 1992; Novic et al. 1984; Walker et al. 1984), others have suggested that schizophrenia patients exhibit a more global deficit in the perception of faces per se (Borod et al. 1993; Feinberg et al. 1986; Gessler et al. 1989; Hellewell et al. 1994; Kerr and Neale 1993; Whittaker et al. 1994). The use of control tasks has been much less common in studies of the perception of vocally expressed emotion. In their study of this domain, Murphy and Cutting (1990) included a control task in which subjects were asked to judge which word in a spoken sentence was emphasized. They found no differences in the performance of patients with schizophrenia and control subjects. Kerr and Neale (1993) used a test of recognition memory for nonsense syllables and, similarly, found no impairment among schizophrenia patients. Because only a small proportion of studies have included control tasks, and these have obtained mixed results, further work—including the development of more appropriately matched control measures—is needed to clarify the precise nature of emotional perception deficits in schizophrenia.

Deficits in Expression

The literature on facial and vocal expression of emotion among patients with schizophrenia suggests that the ability to express emotions may also be disturbed in this disorder. In studies of facial expression, subjects are typically exposed to affective stimuli and their facial expressions are then rated using one of several coding systems. Numerous studies have shown decreased facial expressiveness among schizophrenia patients compared with control subjects during emotion-eliciting films (H. Berenbaum and Oltmanns 1992; Blanchard et al. 1994; Kring et al. 1993; F. Schneider et al. 1990) or emotion-eliciting interviews (Gaebel and Wölwer 1992; Pitman et al. 1987; F. Schneider et al. 1990), as well as in tasks in which subjects are explicitly asked to imitate a particular emotion (Borod et al. 1989, 1990; Braun et al. 1991; Gaebel and Wölwer 1992). Studies of vocal expressiveness have obtained similar results, with schizophrenia patients showing impairment relative to control subjects when asked to read sentences in a particular emotional tone (Borod et al. 1989, 1990; Murphy and Cutting 1990; Whittaker et al. 1994) and also when rated on spontaneous vocal expressivity during an emotion-eliciting interview (Haskins et al. 1995). However, most of the studies examining facial and vocal expression lacked important controls. In particular, measures of subjective emotional experience have not been examined concurrently with measures of emotional expression. If subjects were not experiencing emotions, then their expression of the expected feelings would be muted or absent. The few studies that used subjective measures to examine facial expression of emotion during emotion-eliciting films found that although the patients with schizophrenia showed diminished expressivity compared with controls, they did not differ from the controls in their self-reports of emotion (H. Berenbaum and Oltmanns 1992; Kring and Neale 1996; Kring et al. 1993). These findings highlight the importance of recognizing that a discrepancy often exists between inner experience and outer signs of emotion.

Correlates of Perceptual and Expressive Deficits

There is clearly a great deal of evidence to support the notion that deficits in both the perception and the expression of emotion exist in schizophrenia; however, several important questions concerning the nature of these deficits have not yet been adequately addressed in the literature. One of the foremost issues is whether these types of affective deficits are specific to schizophrenia. A number of studies of affective deficits have included patients with depressive disorders as a psychiatric control group. In the area of perception of facially expressed emotion, some researchers have demonstrated that schizophrenia patients are relatively more impaired than depressed patients, at least on some kinds of tasks (Bellack et al. 1992; Borod et al. 1990; Cutting 1981; Feinberg et al. 1986; Gaebel and Wölwer 1992; Heimberg et al. 1992; Walker et al. 1984). However, on other kinds of tasks, sometimes within the same studies, researchers have failed to find such differences (Borod et al. 1990; Walker et al. 1984; Zuroff and Colussy 1986). Typically, researchers have found that whereas schizophrenia patients show greater deficits than do depressed patients on discrimination tasks (e.g., deciding which of two faces reveals a certain emotion), there are no differences between the groups on labeling tasks (e.g., selecting an emotional label from a number of alternatives to describe a single face). Another important question in this area is whether patients with different subtypes of schizophrenia differ in their performance of perception-of-emotion tasks. Several studies have found that paranoid schizophrenia patients are significantly more accurate than nonparanoid patients on such tasks (Kline et al. 1992; Lewis and Garver 1995). These findings are consistent with the idea that subgroups of schizophrenia patients may differ in terms of their affective functioning—and thus, that this domain of psychopathology may have validity as a way of distinguishing subtypes of the disorder.

Although there is a moderate degree of consensus in the literature concerning differences between schizophrenia patients and depressed patients in the perception of facially expressed emotion, the situation is less clear for the perception of vocally expressed emotion. Borod and colleagues (1990) found that schizophrenia patients were more impaired than depressed patients on a vocal discrimination task but not on a vocal labeling task. Similarly, Murphy and Cutting (1990) found that patients with schizophrenia were not more impaired than either manic patients or depressed patients on a vocal labeling task. While, collectively, these results seem to parallel the findings on perception of facially expressed emotion; however, like those results, they must be viewed with caution until further replication with adequate controls have been reported.

Another important issue in the areas of emotional perception and expression is whether the observed deficits among patients with schizophrenia are associated with negative symptoms. Given that the negative symptoms of schizophrenia have been conceptualized in part as deficits in normal emotional functioning, it might be expected that impairments in emotional perception and expression would be strongly associated with such symptoms. Only a handful of studies have examined this question, and their findings provide no clear consensus. Associations have been noted between various measures of negative symptoms and deficits in the perception of facially expressed emotion (Gaebel and Wölwer 1992; Heimberg et al. 1992), in the perception of vocally expressed emotion (Haskins et al. 1995), in facial expressiveness (H. Berenbaum and Oltmanns 1992; Gaebel and Wölwer 1992; Kring et al. 1994), and in vocal expressiveness (Kring et al. 1994). However, low or nonsignificant correlations have also been reported in the literature (Blanchard et al. 1994; Gaebel and Wölwer 1992; Lewis and Garver 1995; Muzekari and Bates 1977; Novic et al 1984). A number of methodological differences in these studies may underlie the discrepancy in results. The studies varied widely in the symptom and dependent measures they used and in their diagnostic methods. In addition, because many of the studies that failed to find significant correlations between negative symptom measures and dependent variables included only a small number of subjects, they may have had inadequate power to detect such relationships. Thus, although there are some indications that affective deficits are related to negative symptomatology, further research in this area is warranted.

A final question that has been addressed in the literature is whether impaired emotional perception and expression in schizophrenia are associated with a particular pattern of neuropsychological deficits. Several studies suggest that right-hemisphere dysfunction may be related to affective deficits in schizophrenia. For example, the work of Borod and colleagues (1989, 1990, 1993) suggests that patients with right-hemisphere damage and schizophrenia patients are similarly impaired relative to nonpsychiatrically ill, psychiatric, and neurological control groups on perception and expression tasks. Mayer and colleagues (1985) found that decreased facial expression among schizophrenia patients was associated with greater right-hemisphere dysfunction, as measured by a variety of neuropsychological tasks. In contrast, Whittaker et al. (1994) reported associations between frontotemporal dysfunction and impaired perception of both facially expressed and vocally expressed emotion. Another study found that decreased facial expression was not significantly correlated with either right-hemisphere or left-hemisphere composite scores derived from a battery of neuropsychological tests (Blanchard et al. 1994). Thus, the few studies that have been conducted in this area report widely varying results. Again, the lack of comparable methodologies among these studies makes such results difficult to interpret and leaves the issue of neuropsychological correlates of affective functioning somewhat unresolved.

The Experience of Emotion

Although performance and behavioral measures have been used to examine the perception and expression of emotion, such measures cannot assess subjective emotional experience, an important aspect of affective functioning. Whereas the examination of emotional experience might seem inherently more difficult or problematic because this domain of functioning relates to inner states, subjective measures may have certain methodological advantages over objective measures. Emotional experience can be examined empirically with simple self-report measures, which may be less vulnerable to potential confounds (e.g., impaired concentration and attention, neuromotor dysfunction, task difficulty) that affect studies on the perception and expression of emotion. In the context of treatment, patient self-reports provide valuable and unique clinical information. Even though patients with schizophrenia may show some impairment in thinking and communication, self-reports of inner emotional states can nonetheless help clinicians to gain a better understanding of their patients and to plan appropriate treatment interventions.

Self-Report Versus Observational Measures

Evidence from the literature on subjective experience in schizophrenia also suggests that this domain may be independent from the more observable aspects of affective functioning. For example, Bleuler (1911/1950) noted that there was often a discrepancy between patients' lack of observable emotional signs and their reports of internal emotional experience. This observation is supported by findings from several recent studies, in which schizophrenia patients exhibited decreased facial expressiveness during exposure to emotion-eliciting films, yet reported experiencing as much positive and negative emotion as nonpsychiatrically ill control subjects did (H. Berenbaum and Oltmanns 1992; Kring and Neale 1996; Kring et al. 1993). Given that widely used rating scales such as the Scale for the Assessment of Negative Symptoms (SANS; Andreasen 1989) and the Positive and Negative Syndrome Scale (PANSS; Kay et al. 1987) are based on both patient reports and interviewer observations, these results have important implications for research on negative symptoms. Combining objective and subjective data on affective functioning could obscure not only the dissociations between these two domains but also the precise meanings of scores on these scales. Most research has used global scores from the SANS and PANSS as measures of negative symptomatology. Such research could be made more conceptually and methodologically precise by instead examining specific symptoms from the overt (e.g., flat affect, monotone speech) and the subjective (e.g., anhedonia) domains when analyzing data. The use of domain-specific measures, such as self-report instruments or detailed ratings of facial expressiveness, would also allow for greater accuracy in research on affective functioning.

Observable emotional signs and patients' subjective emotional experience differ in their power to predict clinical outcome. For example, several follow-up studies have found that self-report measures of distress are more predictive of relapse (Blanchard et al. 1992; Hirsch and Jolley 1989; Hogarty et al. 1979; Schooler et al. 1980) and of suicide (Cohen et al. 1990) than are clinician-rated measures. These studies suggest that self-report instruments may capture a different aspect of emotional functioning than do observer ratings. Comparisons of self-report and clinician-rated measures of various domains of emotion (e.g., depression, anxiety, negative symptoms) have often found a lack of association between them (Blanchard et al. 1992; Jaeger et al. 1990; Craig and Van Natta 1976; Lindenmayer et al. 1992; Penn et al. 1994). A few studies, however, have obtained significant correlations between self-ratings and observer ratings of depression (Addington et al. 1993; Faustman et al. 1989). Studies comparing self- and observer ratings vary widely in terms of their methodologies (e.g., domain of emotion being examined, instruments used, sample sizes). Nonetheless, collectively, these results suggest that there can be a large discrepancy between the inner and outer signs of emotion in schizophrenia and that subjective assessments are more sensitive in detecting emotional experience than observational techniques.

These kinds of differences between the inner and outer signs of emotion can have tremendous clinical significance. Patients who seem to lack emotion (e.g., who lack facial expressions, have monotone or impoverished speech, display little body language, or are socially withdrawn) may appear this way for numerous reasons. Such symptoms may be secondary to other distinguishable causes, such as paranoia, depression, or medication side effects, or they may be primary, as is the case for patients with the deficit syndrome.

The complexity of this issue is illustrated in the following case vignette.

With a 15-year history of schizophrenia with multiple hospitalizations and an equally long track record of apathy and flattened affect, Mr. H, a 36-year-old man, seemed the archetypal deficit syndrome patient. Treatment with several new atypical antipsychotics aimed at alleviating negative symptoms was not making a dent in his obvious loss of affect. He seemed unconcerned about—even indifferent to—the treatment failures, providing further evidence for the negative symptom subtype diagnosis he had been given.

But, in fact, Mr. H was depressed and probably had been suffering from a major depressive disorder for nearly a year. Although he clearly had negative symptoms stemming from schizophrenia, the severity of the negative syndrome was actually accounted for by his depression. His depressive symptoms only became apparent over the course of several months, during which he was involved in a research study. The research interviewer who evaluated Mr. H independently from the clinical team noted that he reported that he had felt angry and demoralized for several weeks. Moreover, he also had been thinking that he would be better off dead. In adherence to protocol, the interviewer informed the clinical staff of what she had learned. The treating therapists were initially incredulous. Mr. H seemed so devoid of emotion that the news that he was feeling angry and demoralized—and that this was leading to hopeless, suicidal thoughts—came as a great surprise.

But how did the research interviewer uncover what Mr. H's psychiatrist, nurse, and social worker had missed? Quite simply, she was required to ask many more questions about his subjective experience than his clinicians, who had no obvious reasons to do so. Mr. H's history and clinical presentation suggested negative, or deficit, symptoms rather than depression. He did not complain of feeling sad or blue. But when the researcher delved deeply into Mr. H's subjective experience, she learned that he did experience emotion, sometimes quite strongly. Rarely, however, did he express what he was feeling. In fact, Mr. H did not suffer from sad or blue moods, but he did experience significant anhedonia. The anhedonia, sleep disturbance, feelings of worthlessness, thoughts of death and suicide, difficulty concentrating, and psychomotor retardation he was experiencing had persisted for more than 8 months, by Mr. H's account. Ultimately, treatment with an antidepressant significantly improved Mr. H's negative symptoms. Although he still showed significant alogia (he described himself as "a man of few words"), he began to enjoy life again.

Outwardly, to the casual observer, the change may not have seemed significant. When depressed, Mr. H had stayed in his room most of the day and never spoke to anyone spontaneously. Now he spent his days out on the ward, listening to his favorite music on a blaring Walkman or watching television. He still rarely spoke to others unless they addressed him first. But inwardly, the difference was like night and day. He looked forward to leaving the hospital and to the weekend visits with his family, and he no longer felt that life was not worth living. With the improvement in negative symptoms, his physician felt confident about taking Mr. H off the atypical neuroleptic he was on and putting him back on depot injections, which had greatly improved his outpatient medication compliance in the past.

As can be seen from Mr. H's case, an assessment of the patient's inner state can provide a valuable clinical clue as to what factors may be underlying negative symptoms, and, consequently, how they should be treated. In other instances, we have seen subjective feelings of paranoia—as well as the apparent negative symptoms caused by such feelings (e.g., withdrawal, asociality)— reduced by appropriate neuroleptic treatment. Thus, assessments of subjective experience can help the clinician to distinguish between different syndromes within schizophrenia and to treat them appropriately.

However, in the case of distinguishing depression within schizophrenia from the deficit syndrome, the subjective experience of both kinds of patients may appear, on the face of it, to be strikingly similar. Both groups may describe a loss of the ability to feel pleasure. Clinicians can differentiate the two by evaluating whether the anhedonia is state related (i.e., depression within schizophrenia) or trait related (i.e., the deficit syndrome). In the latter case, one would expect to see a more global loss of the ability to feel emotion—that is, the loss of both positive and negative emotional experiences—and not just a loss of the ability to feel pleasure.

Anhedonia

Anhedonia in patients with schizophrenia has been studied empirically, and the literature on this symptom is also relevant to the question raised earlier— that is, of whether a subgroup of patients with negative symptoms lack the capacity to experience emotion fully (for a review, see Ettenberg 1993). As mentioned at the beginning of this chapter, early theoretical formulations (e.g., Bleuler 1911/1950; Kraepelin 1919/1971) viewed anhedonia as a fundamental symptom of schizophrenia. This conceptualization is supported by more recent research, which shows that patients with schizophrenia score higher on anhedonia scales than do control subjects (Brown et al. 1979; Chapman et al. 1976; C. G. Watson et al. 1970). However, these results do not suggest that all patients with schizophrenia are anhedonic, as would be predicted by the genetic predisposition theories of Meehl (1962, 1975) and Rado (1956). For example, Chapman et al. (1976) found that only one-third of their sample of patients with schizophrenia ($n = 121$) scored in the anhedonic range on their Scales for Physical and Social Anhedonia. It is also clear that anhedonia is not specific to schizophrenia. Anhedonia is also prominent among individuals with depressive disorders (Clark and Fawcett 1987; Fawcett et al. 1983; Harrow et al. 1977; MacPhillamy and Lewinsohn 1974; Silverstone 1991). However, anhedonia among schizophrenia patients is not necessarily the result of depression. Chapman et al. (1976) found no association between anhedonia scores and measures of depression in their sample of schizophrenia patients, suggesting that anhedonia can be independent of depressive symptoms in schizophrenia. Although anhedonia is neither a necessary nor a sufficient condition for the development of schizophrenia, it has been found to be a prominent symptom in at least a subgroup of schizophrenia patients. We have suggested in this chapter is that deficits in the ability to experience emotion, such as anhedonia, might underlie deficit or primary negative symptoms in a subgroup of patients. This idea is supported by the finding that patients with the deficit syndrome report greater physical and social anhedonia than do nondeficit patients (Kirkpatrick and Buchanan 1990).

The presence of anhedonia may have significant consequences. It has been hypothesized that anhedonia may result from a deficiency in the brain's reward or reinforcement systems (Meehl 1962, 1975; see Ettenberg 1989 and Wise 1982 for reviews). A relationship between negative or deficit symptoms and deficits in the reward system is supported by evidence that schizophrenia patients with more severe negative symptoms have lower rates of substance abuse than do those with less severe symptoms (Horcajadas et al. 1997; Lysaker et al. 1994). Similar results have been obtained with deficit syndrome patients (Kirkpatrick et al. 1996). Disturbance of positive reinforcement circuits might also account for other negative symptoms, such as apathy, avolition, asociality, and flat affect. Apathy, or emotional indifference, has been assessed with the Scale for Emotional Blunting (SEB; Abrams and Taylor 1978) in a detailed way that emphasizes the subjective nature of this deficit. The SEB includes four "indifference" items, three of which are based on the patient's self-report (Lack of Affection for Family, Unconcern for Own Present Situation, and Unconcern for Own Future) and one of which is based on observation (Indifference to Surroundings). A factor analytic study of the SEB found that these indifference items—especially unconcern for one's own present situation and for one's own future—formed a separate factor (S. A. Berenbaum et al. 1987). Interestingly, the authors labeled this the Avolition factor, implying that diminished emotional experience underlies avolition. This Avolition factor discriminated patients with schizophrenia from patients with depressive disorders, whereas the Emotional Expression factor did not. Although the Avolition factor of the SEB does include a behavioral component, these results nonetheless suggest that subjective reports of diminished emotional experience are conceptually and methodologically useful for distinguishing between schizophrenia-related anhedonia and depression-related anhedonia.

While differences in emotional experience may distinguish between anhedonia as it is manifested in schizophrenia and anhedonia as it is manifested in depression, distinguishing between anhedonia within schizophrenia and depression within schizophrenia is a more complicated matter. Numerous authors have described the difficulty of differentiating negative symptoms from depression in patients with schizophrenia (Knights and Hirsch 1981; Malla 1995; McGlashan and Fenton 1992; Pogue-Geile and Harrow 1984; Prosser et al. 1987; Zubin 1985). As mentioned earlier, a schizophrenic patient with the deficit syndrome and a schizophrenic patient who is depressed may have highly similar presentations in terms of diminished emotional experience. One would expect, however, that such patients would show highly different treatment responses. For example, the anhedonia of the depressed schizophrenic patient would decrease in response to treatment with a selective serotonin reuptake inhibitor (SSRI), while that of the deficit patient would remain unchanged. Although research to date has not specifically examined the treatment response of anhedonia in depressed schizophrenia patients versus deficit syndrome schizophrenia patients, several authors have examined whether negative symptoms more generally are responsive to treatment with SSRIs. These studies have obtained mixed results, with some demonstrating a reduction in negative symptoms when an SSRI is used (Goff et al. 1990, 1995; Silver and Shmugliakov 1998; Spina et al. 1994; Thakore et al. 1996) and others finding no such improvement (Buchanan and Gold 1996; Buchanan et al. 1996; Lee et al. 1998; Taiminen et al. 1997). These conflicting results may be due to a number of confounding factors, such as failure to distinguish between primary and secondary negative symptoms and use of different antipsychotic medications across studies. Further research is needed to address these issues as well as to examine more specifically whether anhedonia is responsive to pharmacological intervention in different subtypes of schizophrenia.

Anhedonia represents a deficit in the ability to experience pleasure or positive emotions. Preliminary evidence also exists for a deficit in the ability to experience negative emotions, at least among a subgroup of patients with schizophrenia. For example, the results of S. A. Berenbaum et al. (1987), discussed earlier, suggest that patients with schizophrenia may show indifference toward both positive and negative experiences. There is also some indication that patients with severe negative symptoms experience fewer negative emotions. In a study examining social anxiety among patients with schizophrenia, Penn et al. (1994) found that higher self-reported anxiety was associated with positive symptoms but not with negative symptoms; only behavioral ratings of anxiety were associated with negative symptomatology. With regard to depression, Kirkpatrick et al. (1994) found that patients with the deficit syndrome reported less-severe depressive symptoms than did nondeficit patients. These results suggest that the experience of negative mood states may also be diminished among patients with primary negative symptoms. The diminishment of both positive and negative emotions in such patients is clinically significant, given that emotional experience plays a key role in motivation. That is, diminished subjective feeling may be associated with impairments in motivated behaviors (e.g., functioning in a socially appropriate way, taking medication, pursuing vocational or other interests).

Research has also begun to examine the subjective experience of negative symptoms per se (Jaeger et al. 1990; Liddle and Barnes 1988; Liddle et al. 1993). The subjective experience of negative symptoms seems to be reported more often among patients with more severe positive and/or depressive symptoms. For example, Jaeger et al. (1990) found that their Subjective Deficit Syndrome Scale (SDSS) was correlated with both depressive and positive symptoms in acute schizophrenia patients, but not with negative symptoms in either acute or chronic schizophrenia patients. Similarly, Liddle and colleagues (1993) found higher Subjective Experience of Deficits in Schizophrenia (SEDS; Liddle and Barnes 1988) scores among depressed schizophrenia patients than among those who were not depressed.

Although only a small amount of work has been done in this area, these results nonetheless seem to indicate that whereas schizophrenia patients with severe negative symptoms may have diminished emotional experience, those patients with positive and affective symptoms "feel more." Although the latter group of patients may at times show diminished subjective feeling as a consequence of positive or depressive symptoms, this lack of feeling is not a stable feature of the illness for them, as it is for deficit patients. Thus, clinically, such patients would present with diminished emotional experience over long periods of time and in a variety of treatment contexts—for example, when unmedicated, on different antipsychotic medications (and on different doses of those medications), and with or without the addition of an SSRI or other antidepressant.

Most of the research on subjective emotional experience discussed thus far has used self-report measures. However, we should note that the use of such instruments in patients with schizophrenia may pose a number of methodological problems. It could be argued that, because of attentional or cognitive impairments, scores on self-report questionnaires may not be representative of a patient's actual subjective experience. In support of this position, a few studies have found that a substantial proportion of schizophrenia patients are unable to complete self-report questionnaires, at least without assistance (Addington et al. 1993; Gerbaldo et al. 1990). It has also been reported that patients with schizophrenia tend to neglect intermediate ratings in favor of the center and extreme positions on self-report scales (Bopp 1955). Some of these difficulties can be minimized by using simpler, more easily understood test formats, such as the true/false format used on the Scales for Physical and Social Anhedonia (Chapman and Chapman 1978; Chapman et al. 1976; Eckblad et al. 1982). Nonetheless, findings based on self-report data should be interpreted with some caution. There are also some methodological concerns relating to interviewer assessments of a patient's subjective experience of negative symptoms, such as those used in the SDSS and the SEDS. Such assessments are obtained in an interpersonal context and thus may be confounded by the social deficits that characterize many patients with schizophrenia (Dworkin 1992).

The Subjective Experience of Pain

In light of these difficulties, alternative ways of conceptualizing and evaluating emotional experience in patients with schizophrenia are needed. In addition to the complexities highlighted above, it has been suggested that affective deficits in schizophrenia may have little or nothing to do with emotion. Rather, affective deficits such as flat affect might result from neuromotor abnormalities (H. Berenbaum and Rotter 1992; Dworkin 1992; Knight and Valner 1993). In light of this alternative conceptualization of affective deficits, a promising line of research is the investigation of pain insensitivity among schizophrenia patients. The study of pain insensitivity allows for the measurement of affective deficits without the potential social/interpersonal and neuromotor confounds inherent in most observer ratings of such deficits (Dworkin 1994). Some have argued that the experience of physical pain is an experience of emotion and, as such, represents an alternative way of examining diminished emotional experience among schizophrenia patients. There is a great deal of evidence to suggest that many schizophrenia patients are less sensitive to physical pain. This phenomenon has been noted clinically ever since the illness was first described (Bleuler 1911/1950; Kraepelin 1919/1971). The prevalence of pain complaints among schizophrenia patients appears to be much lower than that among patients with other psychiatric disorders (Delaplaine et al. 1978; Merskey 1965; Spear 1967; G. D. Watson et al. 1981). There are also numerous reports in the literature that patients with schizophrenia appear to have a reduced sensitivity to pain in a wide variety of conditions, such as bone fractures (Fishbain 1982; Marchand et al. 1959), burns (Shattock 1950), peptic ulcers (Ehrentheil 1957; Hussar 1968; Marchand et al. 1959; West and Hecker 1952), cancer (Talbott and Linn 1978), and heart disease (Hussar 1965, 1966; Lieberman 1955; Marchand 1955; Vanderkamp 1970). Pain insensitivity among schizophrenia patients has also been demonstrated experimentally with the use of a variety of painful stimuli (e.g., thermal, electrical, pin-prick; see Dworkin 1994 for a review).

The experience of pain involves both sensory and emotional aspects. Using methods that distinguish between these different aspects of pain, Dworkin et al. (1993) found that patients with schizophrenia showed significant sensory impairment in discriminating painful thermal stimuli compared with controls. Contrary to prediction, schizophrenia patients as a group did not differ from control subjects in their reports of pain (a measure reflecting subjective experience). However, when the data were examined correlationally, it was found that a higher criterion for the report of pain (i.e., a more "stoical" response to pain) was associated with less-intense emotional experience on a separate task assessing self-reported emotional experience of humor. Moreover, more stoical responses to pain were also associated with greater affective flattening (as measured by the SANS). Collectively, these results suggest that the patients studied had both sensory and emotional deficits. In addition, these findings provide evidence that at least some patients with schizophrenia appear to have a diminished experience of pain that is associated with an affective deficit.

Conclusions

In this chapter we have argued that diminished emotional experience is an independent aspect of affective functioning that is distinguishable from the more easily observable signs of emotion. The assessment of emotional experience has clinical utility as well as certain methodological advantages for studies of negative symptoms in schizophrenia. More research is needed to replicate the findings outlined above. In addition, potential confounds, such as medication effects and cognitive impairments, require examination. These remain important directions for future work.

Given the indications that diminished emotional experience characterizes a subset of patients with schizophrenia, it seems reasonable to hypothesize that this deficit may be associated with particular clinical features. That is, lack of emotional experience may define a distinct syndrome in schizophrenia, the clinical value of which is obvious. In this context, a promising area of investigation is the relationship between diminished emotional experience and the deficit syndrome. One could argue that diminished emotional experience is a deficit or primary negative symptom that is reflected in a number of other symptoms, such as apathy, amotivation, avolition, and flat affect. That is, diminished emotional experience may underlie these deficits in behavior, feeling, and motivation. Research to date on the deficit syndrome has not specifically addressed this issue. The criteria for the deficit syndrome include both items related to the patient's diminished emotional experience (e.g., "curbing of interest" and "diminished sense of purpose" and guidelines regarding clinical judgment of outward emotional signs (e.g., restricted affect, diminished emotional range [Carpenter et al. 1988]). In other words, the deficit syndrome criteria appear to represent a combination of deficits in emotional experience and expression. Future research should focus on determining the relationships among these various affective disturbances and deficit symptoms to illuminate whether impairments in subjective emotional functioning underlie other, more observable impairments.

Another direction for future research concerns other clinical and prognostic features that appear to be related to diminished emotional experience. Elsewhere, we have suggested that emotional functioning represents an important component of insight among patients with schizophrenia (Amador et al. 1991, 1994). Poor insight, or lack of awareness of the signs and symptoms of the illness, of their consequences, and of the need for treatment, is prevalent among these patients and has important implications for the etiology and treatment of schizophrenia (for reviews of this literature, see Amador et al.

1991 and Ghaemi and Pope 1994). Previously, we noted that lack of awareness of illness in neurological disorders, or *anosognosia*, shares many striking similarities with unawareness phenomena in schizophrenia, which suggests the possibility of important phenomenological and etiological parallels between the two (Amador et al. 1991). Babinski (1914) was the first to describe anosognosia, which has been most frequently observed in patients with hemiplegia and hemianopia following stroke. Babinski also described *anosodiaphoria*, or emotional indifference toward one's impairment. Regarding the latter of these components, Gerstmann (1942) observed that when anosognostic patients are shown the affected limb, they often regard it with indifference, indicating not only that they lack awareness of the impairment but also that they have no emotional reaction to it. The evidence reviewed in this chapter suggests that emotional indifference may also exist among certain patients with schizophrenia, and given the similarities of unawareness phenomena in brain-damaged patients and patients with schizophrenia, it seems reasonable to hypothesize that such emotional deficits may represent an important component of lack of insight.

We recently completed two studies (X. F. Amador, M. Friedman M, B. Kirkpatrick, L. Marcinico, S. A. Yale, "Insight in Deficit and Nondeficit Forms of Schizophrenia" [manuscript in preparation, June 2000]; Kasapis et al. 1995) in which we addressed this question by examining the relationships between emotional experience, insight, and deficit symptoms. In the first of these studies, we reported data—replicating findings of an earlier report (Young et al. 1993)—indicating that frontal lobe dysfunction underlies deficits in these areas (Kasapis et al. 1995). We also found that the deficit syndrome and deficit symptoms are strongly correlated with impairment in illness awareness in patients with schizophrenia (Amador et al., manuscript in preparation, June 2000). Preliminary evidence from the insight (Bear 1982; Geschwind 1965; Kasapis et al. 1995; Koehler et al. 1986; McGlynn and Schacter 1989; Young et al. 1993), affect (Borod et al. 1989, 1990, 1993; Mayer et al. 1985; Whittaker et al. 1994), and deficit syndrome (Buchanan et al. 1990; Tamminga et al. 1992) literatures are also consistent with this position. The co-occurrence of poor insight, deficit symptomatology, and diminished emotional experience supports the notion of a distinct syndrome in schizophrenia.

The existence of such a syndrome, with descriptive and predictive validity, would seem to have important implications for diagnosis and treatment. Although a number of recent studies have examined whether the deficit syndrome can be treated pharmacologically (Pelissolo et al. 1996; Suzuki et al.

1996), to our knowledge, no studies to date have specifically examined whether diminished emotional experience in deficit patients responds to such treatments. We suspect that, given the poor prognosis associated with the other aspects of this syndrome (i.e., lack of insight, deficit symptoms, and cognitive impairments), diminished emotional experience may represent a treatment-resistant feature of the illness in these patients—at least with currently available treatments. This idea is supported in our clinical experience, in which we have seen deficit patients whose outward negative symptoms—flat affect, decreased eye contact, monotonous speech, and alogia—improved with treatment with atypical neuroleptics such as risperidone, clozapine, and olanzapine. However, although their affect appeared brighter, these patients still reported a diminished inner state (e.g., not being interested in or upset by much of anything, feeling neither happy or sad). This kind of differential treatment response of inner and outer signs of emotion remains an important area for future research and clinical attention.

References

Abrams R, Taylor MA: A rating scale for emotional blunting. Am J Psychiatry 135:226–229, 1978

Addington D, Addington J, Maticka-Tyndale E: Rating depression in schizophrenia: a comparison of a self-report and an observer report scale. J Nerv Ment Dis 181:561–565, 1993

Amador XF, Strauss DH, Yale SA, et al: Awareness of illness in schizophrenia. Schizophr Bull 17:113–132, 1991

Amador XF, Flaum M, Andreasen NC, et al: Awareness of illness in schizophrenia and schizoaffective and mood disorders. Arch Gen Psychiatry 51:826–836, 1994

American Psychiatric Association: Diagnostic and Statistical Manual of Mental Disorders, 3rd Edition, Revised. Washington, DC, American Psychiatric Association, 1987

American Psychiatric Association: Diagnostic and Statistical Manual of Mental Disorders, 4th Edition. Washington, DC, American Psychiatric Association, 1994

Andreasen NC: The Scale for the Assessment of Negative Symptoms (SANS): conceptual and theoretical foundations. Br J Psychiatry 155 (suppl 7):49–58, 1989

Babinski MJ: Contribution a l'etude des troubles mentaux dans l'hemiplegieorganique cerebale (anosognosie) [Contribution to the study of mental disturbance in organic cerebral hemiplegia (anosognosia)]. Rev Neurol (Paris) 12:845–888, 1914

Bear DM: Hemispheric specialization and neurology of emotion. Arch Neurol 40:195–202, 1982

Bellack AS, Mueser KT, Wade JH, et al: The ability of schizophrenics to perceive and cope with negative affect. Br J Psychiatry 160:473–480, 1992

Berenbaum H, Oltmanns TF: Emotional experience and expression in schizophrenia and depression. J Abnorm Psychol 101:37–44, 1992

Berenbaum H, Rotter A: The relationship between spontaneous facial expressions of emotion and voluntary control of facial muscles. Journal of Nonverbal Behavior 16:179–190, 1992

Berenbaum SA, Abrams R, Rosenberg S, et al: The nature of emotional blunting: a factor-analytic study. Psychiatry Res 20:57–67, 1987

Bilder RM, Mukherjee S, Rieder RO, et al: Symptomatic and neuropsychological components of defect states. Schizophr Bull 11:409–419, 1985

Blanchard JJ, Mueser KT, Bellack AS: Self- and interview-rated negative mood states in schizophrenia: their convergence and prediction of thought disturbance. Journal of Psychopathology, and Behavioral Assessment 14:277–291, 1992

Blanchard JJ, Kring AM, Neale JM: Flat affect in schizophrenia: A test of neuropsychological models. Schizophr Bull 20:311–325, 1994

Bleuler E: Dementia Praecox or the Group of Schizophrenias (1911). Translated by Zinkin J. New York, International Universities Press, 1950

Bopp J: A quantitative semantic analysis of word association in schizophrenia. Dissertation Abstracts 15:2292, 1955

Borod JC, Alpert M, Brozgold A, et al: A preliminary comparison of flat affect schizophrenics and brain-damaged patients on measures of affective processing. J Commun Disord 22:93–104, 1989

Borod JC, Welkowitz J, Alpert M, et al: Parameters of emotional processing in neuropsychiatric disorders: conceptual issues and a battery of tests. J Commun Disord 23:247–271, 1990

Borod JC, Martin CC, Alpert M, et al: Perception of facial emotion in schizophrenic and right brain-damaged patients. J Nerv Ment Dis 181:494–502, 1993

Braun C, Bernier S, Proulx R, et al: A deficit of primary affective facial expression independent of bucco-facial dyspraxia in chronic schizophrenics. Cognition and Emotion 5:147–159, 1991

Brown SL, Sweeney DR, Schwartz GE: Differences between self-reported and observed pleasure in depression and schizophrenia. J Nerv Ment Dis 167:410–415, 1979

Buchanan RW, Gold JM: Negative symptoms: diagnosis, treatment and prognosis. Int Clin Psychopharmacol 11 (suppl 2):3–11, 1996

Buchanan RW, Kirkpatrick B, Heinrichs DW, et al: Clinical correlates of the deficit syndrome of schizophrenia. Am J Psychiatry 147:290–294, 1990

Buchanan RW, Kirkpatrick B, Bryant N, et al: Fluoxetine augmentation of clozapine treatment in patients with schizophrenia. Am J Psychiatry 153:1625–1627, 1996

Carpenter WT Jr, Heinrichs DW, Wagman AMI: Deficit and nondeficit forms of schizophrenia: the concept. Am J Psychiatry 145:578–583, 1988

Chapman LJ, Chapman JP: Revised Physical Anhedonia Scale. Unpublished test, 1978

Chapman LJ, Chapman JP, Raulin ML: Scales for Physical and Social Anhedonia. J Abnorm Psychol 85:374–382, 1976

Clark DC, Fawcett J: Anhedonia, hypohedonia and pleasure capacity in major depressive disorders, in Anhedonia and Affect Deficit States. Edited by Clark DC, Fawcett J. New York, PMA, 1987, pp 51–63

Cohen LJ, Test MA, Brown RL: Suicide and schizophrenia: data from a prospective community treatment study. Am J Psychiatry 147:602–607, 1990

Craig TJ, Van Natta PA: Recognition of depressed affect in hospitalized psychiatric patients: staff and patient perceptions. Diseases of the Nervous System 37:561–566, 1976

Cramer P, Weegmann M, O'Neill M: Schizophrenia and the perception of emotions: how accurately do schizophrenics judge the emotional states of others? Br J Psychiatry 155:225–228, 1989

Cramer P, Bowen J, O'Neill M: Schizophrenics and social judgement: why do schizophrenics get it wrong? Br J Psychiatry 160:481–487, 1992

Cutting J: Judgement of emotional expression in schizophrenia. Br J Psychiatry 139:1–6, 1981

Delaplaine R, Ifabumuyi OI, Merskey H, et al: Significance of pain in psychiatric hospital patients. Pain 4:361–366, 1978

Dougherty FE, Bartlett ES, Izard CE: Responses of schizophrenics to expressions of the fundamental emotions. J Clin Psychol 30:243–246, 1974

Dworkin RH: Affective deficits and social deficits in schizophrenia: what's what? Schizophr Bull 18:59–64, 1992

Dworkin RH: Pain insensitivity in schizophrenia: a neglected phenomenon and some implications. Schizophr Bull 20:235–248, 1994

Dworkin RH, Clark WC, Lipsitz JD, et al: Affective deficits and pain insensitivity in schizophrenia. Motivation and Emotion 17:245–276, 1993

Eckblad M, Chapman LJ, Chapman JP, Mishlove M: The Revised Social Anhedonia Scale. Madison, WI, University of Wisconsin, 1982

Ehrentheil OF: Common medical disorders rarely found in psychotic patients: rarity of hay fever, asthma, and rheumatoid arthritis in contrast to relative frequency of duodenal ulcer in a psychiatric hospital. Archives of Neurology and Psychiatry 77:178–186, 1957

Ettenberg A: Dopamine, neuroleptics and reinforced behavior. Neurosci Biobehav Rev 30:309–317, 1989

Ettenberg A: Anhedonia, in Symptoms of Schizophrenia. Edited by Costello CG. New York, Wiley, 1993, pp 121–144

Faustman WO, Moses JA Jr, Csernansky JG, et al: Correlations between the MMPI and the Brief Psychiatric Rating Scale in schizophrenic and schizoaffective patients. Psychiatry Res 28:135–143, 1989

Fawcett J, Clark DC, Scheftner WA, et al: Assessing anhedonia in psychiatric patients: the pleasure scales. Arch Gen Psychiatry 40:79–84, 1983

Feighner JP, Robins E, Guze SB, et al: Diagnostic criteria for use in psychiatric research. Arch Gen Psychiatry 26:57–83, 1972

Feinberg TE, Rifkin A, Schaffer C, et al: Facial discrimination and emotional recognition in schizophrenia and affective disorders. Arch Gen Psychiatry 43:276–279, 1986

Fenton WS, McGlashan TH: Testing systems for assessment of negative symptoms in schizophrenia. Arch Gen Psychiatry 49:179–184, 1992

Fenton WS, McGlashan TH: Antecedents, symptom progression, and long-term outcome of the deficit syndrome in schizophrenia. Am J Psychiatry 151:351–356, 1994

Fishbain DA: Pain insensitivity in psychosis. Ann Emerg Med 11:630–632, 1982

Gaebel W, Wölwer W: Facial expression and emotional face recognition in schizophrenia and depression. Eur Arch Psychiatry Clin Neurosci 242:46–52, 1992

Gerbaldo H, de las Carreras C, Osuna A, et al: Self-reports in chronic schizophrenic patients with primary negative symptoms: preliminary results. Pharmacopsychiatry 23:195–197, 1990

Gerstmann J: Problem of imperception of disease and of impaired body territories with organic lesions. Relation to body scheme and its disorders. Archives of Neurology and Psychiatry 48:890–913, 1942

Geschwind N: Disconnection syndromes in animals and man. Brain 88:237–294, 585–644, 1965

Gessler S, Cutting J, Frith CD, et al: Schizophrenic inability to judge facial emotion: a controlled study. Br J Clin Psychol 28:19–29, 1989

Ghaemi SN, Pope HG Jr: Lack of insight in psychotic and affective disorders: a review of empirical studies. Harv Rev Psychiatry 2:22–33, 1994

Goff DC, Brotman AW, Waites M, et al: Trial of fluoxetine added to neuroleptics for treatment-resistant schizophrenic patients. Am J Psychiatry 147:492–494, 1990

Goff DC, Midha KK, Sadrid-Segal O, et al: A placebo-controlled trial of fluoxetine added to neuroleptic in patients with schizophrenia. Psychopharmacology (Berl) 117:417–423, 1995

Green M, Walker E: Neuropsychological performance and positive and negative symptoms. J Abnorm Psychol 94:460–469, 1985

Harrow M, Grinker RR Sr, Holzman P, et al: Anhedonia and schizophrenia. Am J Psychiatry 134:794–797, 1977

Haskins B, Shutty MS Jr, Kellogg E: Affect processing in chronically psychotic patients: development of a reliable assessment tool. Schizophr Res 15:291–297, 1995

Heimberg C, Gur RE, Erwin RJ, et al: Facial emotion discrimination, III: behavioral findings in schizophrenia. Psychiatry Res 42:253–265, 1992

Hellewell JSE, Connell J, Deakin JFW: Affect judgement and facial recognition memory in schizophrenia. Psychopathology 27:255–261, 1994

Hirsch SR, Jolley AG: The dysphoric syndrome in schizophrenia and its implications for relapse. Br J Psychiatry 155 (suppl 5):46–50, 1989

Hogarty GE, Schooler NR, Ulrich R, et al: Fluphenazine and social therapy in the aftercare of schizophrenic patients. Arch Gen Psychiatry 36:1283–1294, 19

Horcajadas F, Calo JJ, Gonzalez MA: Drug use and dependence in schizophrenia. Actas Luso-Espanolas de Neurologia, Psiquiatria y Ciencias Afines 25:379–389, 1997

Hussar AE: Coronary heart disease in chronic schizophrenia patients: a clinicopathologic study. Circulation 31:919–929, 1965

Hussar AE: Leading causes of death in institutionalized chronic schizophrenic patients: a study of 1,275 autopsy protocols. J Nerv Ment Dis 142:45–57, 1966

Hussar AE: Peptic ulcer in long-term institutionalized schizophrenic patients. Psychosom Med 30:374–377, 1968

Jaeger J, Bitter I, Czobor P, et al: The measurement of subjective experience in schizophrenia: the Subjective Deficit Syndrome Scale. Compr Psychiatry 31:216–226, 1990

Kane JM: Treatment-resistant schizophrenic patients. J Clin Psychiatry 57 (suppl 9):35–40, 1996

Kane JM, Freeman HL: Towards more effective antipsychotic treatment. Br J Psychiatry Suppl 25:22–31, 1994

Kasapis C, Amador XF, Yale SA, et al: Poor insight in schizophrenia: neuropsychological and defensive aspects (abstract). Schizophr Res 15:123, 1995

Kay SR, Fiszbein A, Opler LA: The Positive and Negative Syndrome Scale (PANSS) for schizophrenia. Schizophr Bull 13:261–276, 1987

Kerr SL, Neale JM: Emotion perception in schizophrenia: specific deficit or further evidence of generalized poor performance? J Abnorm Psychol 102:312–318, 1993

Kinon BJ, Kane JM, Chakos M, et al: Possible predictors of neuroleptic-resistant schizophrenic relapse: influence of negative symptoms and acute extrapyramidal side effects. Psychopharmacol Bull 29:365–369, 1993

Kirkpatrick B, Buchanan RW: Anhedonia and the deficit syndrome of schizophrenia. Psychiatry Res 31:25–30, 1990

Kirkpatrick B, Buchanan RW, Breier A, et al: Depressive symptoms and the deficit syndrome of schizophrenia. J Nerv Ment Dis 182:452–455, 1994

Kirkpatrick B, Amador XF, Yale SA, et al: The deficit syndrome in the DSM-IV field trial, I: alcohol and other drug abuse. Schizophr Res 20:69–77, 1996

Kline JS, Smith JE, Ellis HC: Paranoid and nonparanoid schizophrenic processing of facially displayed affect. J Psychiatr Res 26:169–182, 1992

Knight RA, Valner JB: Affective deficits in schizophrenia, in Symptoms of Schizophrenia. Edited by Costello CG. New York, Wiley, 1993, pp 145–200

Knights A, Hirsch SR: "Revealed" depression and drug treatment for schizophrenia. Arch Gen Psychiatry 38:806–811, 1981

Koehler PJ, Endtz LJ, Te Velde J, et al: Aware or non-aware: on the significance of awareness for the localization of the lesion responsible for homonymous hemianopia. J Neurol Sci 75:255–262, 1986

Kraepelin E: Dementia Praecox and Paraphrenia (1919). Translated by Barclay RM. Huntingdon, NY, RE Krieger, 1971

Kring AM, Neale JM: Do schizophrenic patients show a disjunctive relationship among expressive, experiential, and psychophysiological components of emotion. J Abnorm Psychol 105:249–257, 1996

Kring AM, Kerr SL, Smith DA, et al: Flat affect in schizophrenia does not reflect diminished subjective experience of emotion. J Abnorm Psychol 102:507–517, 1993

Kring AM, Alpert M, Neale JM, et al: A multimethod, multichannel assessment of affective flattening in schizophrenia. Psychiatry Res 54:211–222, 1994

Lee MS, Kim YK, Lee SK, et al: A double-blind study of adjunctive sertraline in haloperidol-stabilized patients with chronic schizophrenia. J Clin Psychopharmacol 18:399–403, 1998

Lewis SF, Garver DL: Treatment and diagnostic subtype in facial affect recognition in schizophrenia. J Psychiatr Res 29:5–11, 1995

Liddle PF: Schizophrenic syndromes, cognitive performance, and neurological dysfunction. Psychol Med 17:49–57, 1987

Liddle PF, Barnes TRE: The subjective experience of deficits in schizophrenia. Compr Psychiatry 29:157–164, 1988

Liddle PF, Barnes TRE, Curson DA, et al: Depression and the experience of psychological deficits in schizophrenia. Acta Psychiatr Scand 88:243–247, 1993

Lieberman AL: Painless myocardial infarction in psychotic patients. Geriatrics 10:579–580, 1955

Lindenmayer JP, Kay SR, Plutchik R: Multivantaged assessment of depression in schizophrenia. Psychiatry Res 42:199–207, 1992

Lysaker P, Bell M, Beam-Goulet J, et al: Relationship of positive and negative symptoms to cocaine abuse in schizophrenia. J Nerv Ment Dis 182:109–112, 1994

MacPhillamy DJ, Lewinsohn PM: Depression as a function of levels of desired and observed pleasure. J Abnorm Psychol 83:651–657, 1974

Malla AK: Negative symptoms and affective disturbance in schizophrenia and related disorders. Can J Psychiatry 40 (suppl 2):55S–59S, 1995

Mandal MK, Palchoudhury S: Decoding of facial affect in schizophrenia. Psychol Rep 56:651–652, 1985

Mandal MK, Palchoudhury S: Identifying the components of facial emotion and schizophrenia. Psychopathology 22:295–300, 1989

Marchand WE: Occurrence of painless myocardial infarction in psychotic patients. N Engl J Med 253:51–55, 1955

Marchand WE, Sarota B, Marble HC, et al: Occurrence of painless acute surgical disorders in psychotic patients. N Engl J Med 260:580–585, 1959

Mayer M, Alpert M, Stastny P, et al: Multiple contributions to clinical presentation of flat affect in schizophrenia. Schizophr Bull 11:420–426, 1985

McGlashan TH, Fenton WS: The positive-negative distinction in schizophrenia: review of natural history validators. Arch Gen Psychiatry 49:63–72, 1992

McGlynn SM, Schacter DL: Unawareness of deficits in neuropsychological syndromes. J Clin Exp Neuropsychol 11:143–205, 1989

Meehl PE: Schizotaxia, schizotypy, and schizophrenia. Am Psychol 17:827–838, 1962

Meehl PE: Hedonic capacity: some conjectures. Bull Menninger Clin 39:295–307, 1975

Merskey H: The characteristics of persistent pain in psychological illness. J Psychosom Res 9:291–298, 1965

Murphy D, Cutting J: Prosodic comprehension and expression in schizophrenia. J Neurol Neurosurg Psychiatry 53:727–730, 1990

Muzekari LH, Bates ME: Judgment of emotion among chronic schizophrenics. J Clin Psychol 33:662–666, 1977

Novic J, Luchins DJ, Perline R: Facial affect recognition in schizophrenia: is there a differential deficit? Br J Psychiatry 144:533–537, 1984

Pelissolo A, Krebs MO, Olie JP: Treatment of negative symptoms in schizophrenia by amisulpride: review of the literature. Encephale 22:215–219, 1996

Penn DL, Hope DA, Spaulding W, et al: Social anxiety in schizophrenia. Schizophr Res 11:277–284, 1994

Pilowsky I, Bassett D: Schizophrenia and the response to facial emotion. Compr Psychiatry 21:236–244, 1980

Pitman RK, Kolb B, Orr SP, et al: Ethological study of facial behavior in nonparanoid and paranoid schizophrenic patients. Am J Psychiatry 144:99–102, 1987

Pogue-Geile MF, Harrow M: Negative and positive symptoms in schizophrenia and depression: a follow-up. Schizophr Bull 10:371–387, 1984

Pogue-Geile MF, Zubin J: Negative symptomatology and schizophrenia: a conceptual and empirical review. International Journal of Mental Health 16:3–45, 1988

Prosser ES, Csernansky JG, Kaplan J, et al: Depression, parkinsonian symptoms, and negative symptoms in schizophrenics treated with neuroleptics. J Nerv Ment Dis 175:100–105, 1987

Rado S: Psychoanalysis of Behavior: Collected Papers. New York, Grüne & Stratton, 1956

Schneider F, Heimann H, Himer W, et al: Computer-based analysis of facial action in schizophrenic and depressed patients. Eur Arch Psychiatry Clin Neurosci 240:67–76, 1990

Schneider K: Clinical Psychopathology. Translated and edited by Hamilton MW. New York, Grune & Stratton, 1959

Schooler NR, Levine J, Severe JB, et al: Prevention of relapse in schizophrenia: an evaluation of fluphenazine decanoate. Arch Gen Psychiatry 37:16–24, 1980

Shattock FM: The somatic manifestations of schizophrenia: a clinical study of their significance. Journal of Mental Science 96:32–142, 1950

Silver H, Shmugliakov N: Augmentation with fluvoxamine but not maprotiline improves negative symptoms in treated schizophrenia: evidence for a specific serotonergic effect from a double-blind study. J Clin Psychopharmacol 18:208–211, 1998

Silverstone PH: Is anhedonia a good measure of depression? Acta Psychiatr Scand 83:249–250, 1991

Smith RC, Chua JW, Lipetsker B, et al: Efficacy of risperidone in reducing positive and negative symptoms in medication-refractory schizophrenia: an open prospective study. J Clin Psychiatry 57:460–466, 1996

Spear FG: Pain in psychiatric patients. J Psychosom Res 11:187–193, 1967

Spina E, De Domenico P, Ruello C, et al: Adjunctive fluoxetine in the treatment of negative symptoms in chronic schizophrenic patients. Int Clin Psychopharmacol 9:281–285, 1994

Spitzer RL, Endicott J, Robins E: Research Diagnostic Criteria for a Selected Group of Functional Disorders, 3rd Edition. New York, New York State Psychiatric Institute and Biometrics Research, 1977

Suzuki E, Kanba S, Koshikawa H, et al: Negative symptoms in nondeficit syndrome respond to neuroleptic treatment with changes in plasma homovanillic acid concentrations. J Psychiatry Neurosci 21:167–171, 1996

Taiminen TJ, Syvalahti E, Saarijarvi S, et al: Citalopram as an adjuvant in schizophrenia: Further evidence for a serotonergic dimension in schizophrenia. Int Clin Psychopharmacol 12:31–35, 1997

Talbott JA, Linn L: Reactions of schizophrenics to life-threatening disease. Psychiatr Q 50:218–227, 1978

Tamminga CA, Thaker GK, Buchanan RW, et al: Limbic system abnormalities identified in schizophrenia using positron emission tomography with fluorodeoxyglucose and neocortical alterations with deficit syndrome. Arch Gen Psychiatry 49: 522–530, 1992

Thakore JH, Berti C, Dinan TG: An open trial of adjunctive sertraline in the treatment of chronic schizophrenia. Acta Psychiatr Scand 94:194–197, 1996

Vanderkamp H: Clinical anomalies in patients with schizophrenia. Experimental Medicine and Surgery 28:291–293, 1970

Walker E, Marwit SJ, Emory E: A cross-sectional study of emotion recognition in schizophrenics. J Abnorm Psychol 89:428–236, 1980

Walker E, McGuire M, Bettes B: Recognition and identification of facial stimuli by schizophrenics and patients with affective disorders. Br J Clin Psychol 23:37–44, 1984

Watson CG, Klett WG, Lotei TW: Toward an operational definition of anhedonia. Psychol Rep 26:371–376, 1970

Watson GD, Chandarana PC, Merskey H: Relationships between pain and schizophrenia. Br J Psychiatry 138:33–36, 1981

West BM, Hecker AO: Peptic ulcer: incidence and diagnosis in psychotic patients. Am J Psychiatry 109:35–37, 1952

Whittaker JF, Connell J, Deakin JFW: Receptive and expressive social communication in schizophrenia. Psychopathology 27:262–267, 1994

Wise RA: Neuroleptics and operant behavior: the anhedonia hypothesis. Behav Brain Sci 5:39–87, 1982

Young DA, Davila R, Scher H: Unawareness of illness and neuropsychological performance in chronic schizophrenia. Schizophr Res 10:117–124, 1993

Zubin J: Negative symptoms: are they indigenous to schizophrenia? Schizophr Bull 11:461–470, 1985

Zuroff DC, Colussy SA: Emotion recognition in schizophrenic and depressed inpatients. J Clin Psychol 42:411–416, 1986

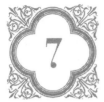

The Family Perspective in the Assessment of Negative Symptom Treatment Efficacy

Dale L. Johnson, Ph.D.

Relatives of people with schizophrenia are familiar with negative symptoms. Positive symptoms can be puzzling, alarming, and often frightening, but medications tend to reduce them to acceptable levels. They are also easier to understand as part of a psychotic process. Negative symptoms have more insidious effects. In a sense, they can be less alarming and more annoying because they overlap with familiar behaviors and may appear to be part of the person's character. They resemble laziness or social reticence, and as such—appearing in American society, which assigns these behaviors low status—they are devalued and even abhorred.

In this chapter, I review three areas of family involvement in the assessment of negative symptoms: 1) assessment of the burden of schizophrenia for families, 2) evaluation of the efficacy of clinical trials, and 3) use of assessment procedures in recovery-oriented interventions.

Assessment of the Burden of Schizophrenia for Families

Large numbers of people with schizophrenia live with relatives, mainly parents, and additional numbers are in regular contact with relatives while living in their own apartments or in group homes. Goldman (1982) estimated that 60% of schizophrenia patients live with relatives. Family members are therefore the single greatest providers of care for people with this illness.

For most of these relatives, the behavior of the person with schizophrenia is a matter of deep concern and the object of close observation. Families are wary of exacerbations of symptoms, knowing that the ill person may become more difficult to live with and even dangerous. They also monitor symptoms closely in order to make changes in the environment that will reduce stress or motivate the person to attempt to accomplish more.

That living with mental illness is to be burdened has been demonstrated often. Burden research has usually examined two types of burden, subjective and objective. *Subjective burden* refers to the reactions of relatives to the behaviors of the ill person. *Objective burden* can be divided into two categories. The first category deals with how the illness interferes with household routines or family relationships. The second type refers to which patient behaviors concern relatives most; that is, what behaviors they worry about or perceive as abnormal (Hoenig 1968; Johnson 1990; Platt 1985).

The assessment of objective burden has not been standardized. In their survey of family burden measures, Schene et al. (1994) identified 21 measures used since 1984. Of these, 7 were designed for use with family members of schizophrenia patients. Although most of these measures include items on symptoms or dysfunctional behaviors, there is little agreement on how to systematically assess these behaviors.

The relative importance of negative symptoms for relatives may be seen in how these symptoms appear when placed in rank order with positive symptoms. Several burden studies have reported results in this way. Thus, Hatfield (1978) reported that family members judged the following behaviors to be disturbing, in rank order (negative symptoms are in **bold** type): **lacks motivation**, handles money poorly, **shows poor grooming and personal care**, has unusual eating and sleeping habits, **forgets to do things**, talks without making sense, argues too much, refuses to take medication, thinks people talk about him/her, hears voices, and breaks and damages things. Spaniol and colleagues (1984) found that concern was greatest for schizophrenic symptoms, depression, **listlessness and low energy**, and aggressiveness. Creer and Wing (1975) conducted a similar survey in the United Kingdom. The behaviors most frequently cited were **social withdrawal, underactivity, lack of conversation**, overactivity, **few leisure interests**, odd ideas, odd behavior, depression, **neglect of appearance**, and odd postures and movements. Lefley's (1987) sample of mental health professionals with a mentally ill family member ranked as very important mood swings, disruption of household routines, social isolation, lack of motivation, poor handling of money, unusual sleep patterns, verbal abuse of others, and refusal to take medication.

Three more-recent studies used methods other than ranking to examine the relative importance of negative symptoms for relatives. Veltro et al. (1994) found that with Italian families, negative symptoms were perceived as most burdensome. This was also the case for families in India, as studied by Gopinath and Chaturvedi (1992). However, positive symptoms presented a greater burden for Malay families (Salleh 1994).

It is obvious from these surveys and others not cited here that the level of objective burden for families is high. The findings seem similar across nations, with essentially the same results in Canada, India, the United Kingdom, and the United States. Actually, however, it is difficult to make direct comparisons of the various studies, because they have differed so much methodologically. Although most of the studies used questionnaires or structured interviews, the format and content of the measures differed.

When burden studies are examined from the perspective of negative symptom assessment, it is apparent that better measures are needed. All of the studies reviewed used crude measures of negative symptoms—that is, they approximated behaviors rated in specific measures such as the Scale for the Assessment of Negative Symptoms (SANS; Andreasen 1989)—and there was little agreement on which measures to use. There did seem to be relatively frequent use of the Social Behaviour Assessment Schedule (SBAS; Platt et al. 1980) (to be discussed later in this chapter); of the measures examined, the SBAS has greatest relevance for negative symptom assessment.

Evaluation of the Effectiveness of Clinical Trials

Medication Trials

A review of the literature reporting efficacy of the newer antipsychotic medications clozapine, risperidone, quetiapine, ziprasidone, and olanzapine makes it clear that this type of evaluation is almost exclusively a matter for patients and provider/researcher staff. Families are rarely if ever included as sources of information in drug efficacy trials. Our review, admittedly not exhaustive, did not find any research that made use of relatives' reports of patient behaviors in drug trials. This is somewhat surprising, given that the newer, atypical antipsychotic medications are often tested in community settings because patients do not stay long in hospitals. Collins et al. (1991) surveyed the drug trial literature for typical antipsychotics and found that 13% of the studies "considered the patient's self-report or ratings of significant others." They concluded that "treatment effectiveness continues to be unidimensional and symptom based. Treatment effectiveness may be obscured when measures of patient functioning, subjective experience, and assessments of significant others are not included with those of symptomatology" (p. 249).

Relatives were included in two medication studies in which the effect of medication on the burden of living with a serious mental illness was examined (Meltzer 1992; Stevens 1973). Both studies found that burden was reduced, but neither study was concerned with the relatives' ratings of the patient's negative symptoms as such.

In the psychopharmacology area, the emphasis in treating psychotic disorders has been on reducing positive symptoms. Furthermore, management of these symptoms has typically taken place in hospitals, where trained nursing staff were on hand to monitor changes in symptom status. With the increased emphasis on negative symptoms and with more patients being treated in the community, symptom monitoring is no longer performed by trained hospital staff. This creates a gap in observation sensitivity, a gap that was partly responsible for a medication research scandal that made national news (Willwerth 1993). In this incident, researchers began treatment of a male patient in a hospital. When the patient's condition improved, he was released to his parents' home. His parents observed his condition, noted deterioration, and reported this to the researchers. Unfortunately, the researchers failed to take the parents' reports seriously, and the patient's condition worsened to a psychotic state. The parents eventually sued the researchers for not providing an adequate informed consent. However, the symptom monitoring process appears to have been as much of the problem as the specifications of the informed consent. If the parents had been included in the monitoring process, trained in the use of observational methods, and encouraged to report on a regular basis, and if the researchers had valued the information provided, the impending crisis might have been detected and averted.

There have been other, similar cases that have not led to media or legal presentations but that are no less serious. Certainly, as clinical trials are extended into communities, members of patients' communities, relatives, {and/ ?}or board-and-care providers will need to be asked to take on assessment responsibilities and be included as members of the evaluation team.

Psychosocial Trials

Medication trials are not the only forms of evaluation that might benefit from relatives' assessments. Family psychoeducation efficacy trials would seem to be prime candidates for the involvement of families. However, trials of the effectiveness of family psychoeducation have only rarely used relatives' assessments of negative symptoms. Of the many trials that have provided family psychoeducation—that is, having the patient and family receive information and training together—only Falloon et al. (1987) and McFarlane et al. (1996) included relatives' ratings of negative symptoms in their evaluation of program efficacy.

Falloon et al. (1987) used seven scales from the SBAS: Household tasks, Leisure activity, Work activity, Decision-making, Friendliness/affection, Everyday conversation, and Outside relationships. Behavior was rated on Impairment and Dissatisfaction. The results over 2 years showed in some detail areas of the patient's life that were affected by the family program and areas that were not. The program had greater effects on performance of household tasks and decision-making than on the other areas measured. However, combining SBAS scores resulted in significant differences favoring the family program. In addition, the measures revealed that 41% of the patients were free of behaviors suggesting negative symptoms at the 24-month follow-up.

McFarlane et al. (1996) used the Social Adjustment Scale III, Family Version (Kreisman et al. 1988), in a comparison of two levels of family-aided assertive community treatment. Results for that study have not yet been reported.

Involvement of the Family in Research and Treatment

That relatives of people with serious mental illnesses should be involved in research and treatment as allies with professionals has been proposed by Johnson (1987) and Kuipers (1993), among others. This partnership is necessitated by the fact that schizophrenia is a long-term and disabling condition, the management of which requires the efforts of many people, not only in hospitals but also in communities.

One of the questions that arises when it is suggested that relatives be asked to provide information in a systematic way is whether they can supply reliable information. Although little is known about this with regard to negative symptom assessment, there is ample evidence of relatives' ability to provide reliable information in other areas. For example, parents are the major source of information in the identification of behavior problems in children (e.g., Barkley 1990). The other main source is teachers. Although agreement between these two sources is low, the difference is more a matter of different perspectives than of interrater reliability. Similar results might be expected from community studies of negative symptoms.

Families rarely receive training in the assessment of symptomatic behaviors. Herz and Melville (1980) have recommended training families and patients to become aware of early signs of relapse. With this identification, steps might be taken to intervene before a full relapse occurs. Relatives can perform this monitoring very well.

Some schizophrenia patients and their families have already learned to use rating scales such as the Brief Psychiatric Rating Scale (BPRS; Lukoff et al. 1986) to monitor symptom levels. Although research is lacking on this use of such instruments, there is no reason why all of the standard symptom scales could not be used with relatives as sources of information. Of course, for reliable, meaningful ratings, family members would require the same kind of training that professional staff receive in use of these measures.

Perhaps the main reason that families are so seldom asked to rate symptom behaviors is that not all patients have relatives living near treatment or research facilities. Locating and involving relatives calls for additional effort and cost. Furthermore, some researchers believe that it is better to have the same trained observers complete ratings. The fact that such observers have very limited exposure to the patients, especially given that patients no longer are hospitalized throughout the study period, is viewed as a problem by many researchers, albeit one that has not yet been solved. It may be time to reexamine assumptions about relatives as sources of systematic information and to develop ways of resolving some of the data collection impediments.

Relatives can be invited to participate in several ways—and the emphasis should be on "invited." Participation should be entirely voluntary. Furthermore, in order to obtain reliable information, family respondents would require training in the use of research measures. Under these conditions, relatives can

- respond to interviews carried out by professional staff,
- complete questionnaires alone, or
- conduct structured interviews such as the BPRS or the Positive and Negative Syndrome Scale (PANSS; Kay et al. 1987).

Assessment of Negative Symptoms

Very few measures of negative symptoms were designed specifically for use by relatives of people with schizophrenia. In addition, although there are many measures of family burden, coping, role functioning, expressed emotion, communication deviance, and other matters pertaining to family members themselves, few measures of relatives' perceptions of the patient's symptom status are available.

Of the scales that have been developed especially for use by relatives, none has a clear focus on negative symptoms. The following scales, however, have some relevance for negative symptom assessment.

The *Social Behaviour Assessment Schedule* (SBAS; Platt et al. 1980) was developed to measure the patient's social behavior and its impact on significant others. A relative who knows the patient well is interviewed. The patient's level of disturbance and social performance are the areas most relevant for assessment of negative symptoms. The SBAS includes ratings of Slowness/Underactivity and Self-Neglect/Poor Hygiene/Poor Grooming. All of the Social Performance subscales appear relevant to negative symptoms: Household Tasks, Spare Time/Leisure Activity, Work/Study, Decision-Making, Friendliness/Affection, Everyday Conversation, and Relationships Outside Family.

Apparently, in the development of the SBAS, reliability of relatives as observers of their patient relatives' behaviors was not determined (Platt et al. 1980). Intraclass correlations for the SBAS subscales ranged from .92 to .99, indicating good reliability. Interrater reliabilities were also high.

The *Social Adjustment Scale III, Family Version* (SAS-III; Kreisman et al. 1988) is an interview designed to be conducted with a relative or significant other. It includes Role Performance, Social Behavior and Role, and Social Interaction variables. Scales that are closest to negative symptoms are Performance Adequacy, Leisure Activities, Interpersonal Relations, Romantic Involvement, Relations With Neighbors, and Self-Care. Reliabilities for the SAS-III are not provided by the scale's authors.

The *Social Functioning Scale* (SFS; Birchwood et al. 1990) was developed for use in family intervention programs. It may be used in either questionnaire or interview form. The scale has 42 items covering seven areas: Withdrawn/Social Engagement, Interpersonal Communication, Independence-Performance, Independence-Competence, Recreation, Prosocial, and Employment/Occupation. Although scores are obtained for each scale, psychometric studies of the SFS indicate that the scales comprise a single factor; thus, the Total score, which has highest reliability, may provide the best measure of social functioning. Birchwood et al. (1990) reported that the correlation between SFS Total score and Present State Examination (PSE; Wing et al. 1974) negative symptoms was .44 ($P < .01$). Barrowclough and Tarrier (1990) found the SFS responsive to change brought about by a family intervention program.

Although these three measures were intended for use with relatives, they were not designed to focus especially on either negative or positive symptoms. Such a measure remains to be developed.

From Relapse Management to Recovery

Most treatment efforts with schizophrenic patients are directed at managing symptoms to prevent relapse. Ever since Kraepelin (1919/1971), mental health professionals have been pessimistic about the long-term prospects for people with this illness, but today there is reason for more optimism. Warner (1985) reviewed 68 longitudinal studies of the course of schizophrenia and concluded that complete recovery occurs in 20%–25% and social recovery occurs in 40%–45% of cases. *Complete recovery* does not mean that the person is "cured," since elements of the illness may remain: rather, it means that the person is able to function in the community without symptom interference.

The negative symptoms of schizophrenia have profound effects on social relations. Lack of social responsiveness and expressiveness mark the schizophrenia patient as different—and uninteresting. As the patient becomes increasingly withdrawn, ordinary routines of interpersonal relationships become disrupted, and other people, including friends and lovers, unsure of a relationship that once seemed predictable and comfortable, may withdraw. Contacts with those people often become less frequent and less satisfactory for the patient. Social networks become smaller and are eventually limited to immediate family (Hamilton et al. 1989). Families may become the patient's last resort as connections to the rest of the social world. They provide for the patient's basic needs, they find the patient and bring him or her back from homelessness, and they take on the burdensome task of seeking professional assistance when their own assistance is rejected by the patient. In the United States there are no legal requirements that families take on these tasks for adult relatives, but they do so nationwide because of the affective ties to and feeling of responsibility for their loved ones.

To date, the most advanced form of family intervention is a set of programs collectively called family psychoeducation. These programs provide information and training—to the family and patient together—on problem-solving and coping skills over a period of time ranging from several months to 2 years. Family psychoeducation, as developed by Leff and associates (1982) in London and elaborated in several other settings (see Lam 1991), has been shown in controlled research to be highly effective in reducing rates of relapse (e.g., at the 2-year follow-up, average program relapse was 28%

compared with 63% for controls) and, in the case of the Southern California project (Falloon et al. 1987), in significantly reducing symptom levels. Through management of environmental stress, people with serious mental illnesses have a more benign course of the illness. This research has laid the groundwork for teaching families how they can help without being too intrusive. The focus has been on preventing or delaying relapse. Now it is time to move ahead to a recovery paradigm. What can be done to promote patient recovery and restore patients to full functioning?

When negative symptoms persist, it is conventional to recommend use of psychosocial interventions such as token economies, social skills training, life skills training, self-instructional training, and problem solving (Slade and Bentall 1989). Suggestions for alternative medications are also made (e.g., Carpenter 1996). It is not usual to suggest that the family or other community caretakers of the patient be encouraged and trained to work to counter negative symptoms. Enlisting family assistance in rehabilitation offers two unique advantages: 1) the activities can continue for years rather than only a few months as is common in clinic-based rehabilitation, and 2) the training would take place in real-life settings, thus making it immediately practical and promoting generalization.

It is envisioned that ongoing assessment of patient symptom status would be part of the long-term recovery-enhancement plan. This use of assessment was described by Gardner and Hunter in their multimodal functional model for treating serious mental illnesses (W. I. Gardner and R. H. Hunter, "The Multimodal Functional Model Enhances Treatment for People With Serious Mental Illness" [unpublished manuscript], August 1995). In this model, a treatment plan is first developed based in part on assessment of the patient's symptom status, social situation, resources, and liabilities. Long- and short-term objectives are then established, and their attainment is assessed with the use of an appropriate battery of measures. Although this model was developed for community mental health center staff, it could be adapted for use with relatives of people with serious mental illnesses. Ongoing assessment is a key part of the process, because family members and the patient need to know where they are and where they have been.

In work with families, the various rehabilitation activities to be undertaken should be directed at negative symptoms and should therefore be those that encourage social interaction, affective arousal, interest in self-improvement, and lengthened span of attention. Such activities might include taking part in community meetings, going to movies, taking community college courses, engaging in regular exercise at a health club, reading newspapers aloud and discussing contents, playing games socially or on computers, participating in Sierra Club hikes, attending art gallery openings, going to athletic events, and so on. The range of activities is unlimited and the choice is based on what is naturally available to the family and community. What makes these different from ordinary family activities is that they are selected to achieve preselected goals, and progress is monitored through the use of rating scales. Activities can be adapted, increased, or broadened to bring about measurable changes. Changes are expected to occur slowly over an extended period.

Recent research in health psychology suggests another way in which families can help to foster recovery. This research has placed emphasis on the relationship of patient and professional in dealing with severe and long-term disorders or illnesses. In the clinician–patient partnership, the clinician is responsible for structuring the course of treatment, and the patient is responsible for carrying out the treatment. Marks (1994) recently described how this partnership works:

> Self-care is a major issue if I have a chronic disease, like diabetes, that requires not just one episode of treatment but permanent, ongoing care, without which I will die. I may have to inject insulin every day, varying the dose according to my response, exercise, and stress; test my urine for sugar and ketones; and carefully monitor my diet. At intervals, the clinician advises me what to do, but in the final analysis it is I who have to carry out the treatment. (p. 20)

The situation Marks describes is much like the situation for people recovering from a serious mental illness.

Marks (1994) went on to show that the outcomes of interventions that require active, ongoing participation by the patient are better if the interventions have certain characteristics, such as close adherence to the prescribed treatment. Such adherence is improved if patients keep records of medication taking, occasions of stress, practice of exercise, and the like.

At present, most professional prescriptions are vague: "take these pills," "go to the psychosocial club," "learn to cope." In contrast, the methods developed by health psychologists are highly specific. It is possible to see that one has achieved something or–if failure is experienced–to know what to do next to improve one's chances of success.

Looking Toward the Future

Accurate assessment of the patient's symptoms in the move toward recovery requires symptom measures that are highly sensitive and ecologically valid (i.e., grounded in real-life behaviors [Bronfenbrenner 1977]). Instruments available at present are not adequate. It is fairly obvious that negative symptoms are present neither in a homogeneous way nor at all times. People with prominent negative symptoms are at times quite expressive and in some situations are motivated to explore new experiences. What is not at all obvious is why, when, and where these symptom changes occur. Are there changes in the environment that result in alleviation of negative symptoms? What can be done to maintain a symptom-free state? Answers to these questions call for a better understanding of the natural course of negative symptoms in the lives of people who have schizophrenia. This, in turn, calls for better assessment measures.

One type of instrument that is needed is an easy-to-use, family-recorded measure of day-to-day behaviors. How do negative symptoms appear in ordinary behavior? Something like the Vineland Adaptive Behavior Scales (Sparrow et al. 1984) may be useful. (The Vineland itself is not appropriate for most adult psychiatric patients.) For example, in assessing the amotivational syndrome, the use of questions such as "Does s/he put dishes in dishwasher without reminding?" could be part of a scale.

Gaining a better understanding of the ordinary appearance of negative symptoms may require strategies such as videotaping of problem-solving or social interactions. The work of Walker and colleagues (1993) on affective expression provides useful suggestions in this regard. Although development of new measures of negative symptoms that are appropriate for use in the community by families will be difficult, such measures will be essential for the expansion of knowledge.

References

Andreasen NC: The Scale for the Assessment of Negative Symptoms (SANS): conceptual and theoretical foundations. Br J Psychiatry 155 (suppl 7):49–58, 1989

Barkley RA: Attention-Deficit Hyperactivity Disorder: A Handbook for Diagnosis and Treatment. New York, Guilford, 1990

Barrowclough C, Tarrier N: Social functioning in schizophrenic patients, I: the effects of expressed emotion and family intervention. Soc Psychiatry Psychiatr Epidemiol 25:125–129, 1990

Birchwood M, Smith J, Cochrane R, et al: The Social Functioning Scale: the development and validation of a new scale of social adjustment for use in family intervention programmes with schizophrenic patients. Br J Psychiatry 157:853–859, 1990

Bronfenbrenner U: Toward an experimental ecology of human development. Am Psychol 32:513–531, 1977

Carpenter WT Jr: Maintenance therapy of persons with schizophrenia. J Clin Psychiatry 57 (suppl 9):10–18, 1996

Collins EJ, Hogan TP, Desai H: Measurement of therapeutic response in schizophrenia: a critical survey. Schizophr Res 5:249–253, 1991

Creer C, Wing JK: Living with a schizophrenic patient. British Journal of Hospital Medicine 14:73–82, 1975

Falloon IRH, McGill CW, Boyd JL, et al: Family management in the prevention of morbidity of schizophrenia: social outcome of a two-year longitudinal study. Psychol Med 17:59–66, 1987

Goldman HH: Mental illness and family burden: a public health perspective. Hospital and Community Psychiatry 33:557–559, 1982

Gopinath PS, Chaturvedi SK: Distressing behaviour of schizophrenics at home. Acta Psychiatr Scand 86:185–188, 1992

Hamilton NG, Ponzoha CA, Cutler DL, et al: Social networks and negative versus positive symptoms of schizophrenia. Schizophr Bull 15:625–633, 1989

Hatfield AB: Psychological costs of schizophrenia to the family. Soc Work 23:355–359, 1978

Herz MI, Melville C: Relapse in schizophrenia. Am J Psychiatry 137:801–805, 1980

Hoenig J: The de-segregation of the psychiatric patient. Proceedings of the Royal Society of Medicine 61:115–120, 1968

Johnson DL: Professional-family collaboration, in Families of the Mentally Ill: Meeting the Challenges. Edited by Hatfield A. San Francisco, CA, Jossey-Bass, 1987, pp 73–80

Johnson DL: The family's experience of living with mental illness, in Families as Allies in Treatment of the Mentally Ill. Edited by Lefley HP, Johnson DL. Washington, DC, American Psychiatric Press, 1990, pp 31–63

Kay SR, Fiszbein A, Opler LA: The Positive and Negative Syndrome Scale (PANSS) for schizophrenia. Schizophr Bull 13:261–276, 1987

Kraepelin E: Dementia Praecox and Paraphrenia (1919). Translated by Barclay RM. Huntingdon, NY, RE Krieger, 1971

Kreisman D, Blumenthal R, Borenstein M, et al: Family attitudes and patient social adjustment in a longitudinal study of outpatient schizophrenics receiving low-dose neuroleptics: the family's view. Psychiatry 51:3–13, 1988

Kuipers L: Family burden in schizophrenia: implications for services. Soc Psychiatry Psychiatr Epidemiol 28:207–210, 1993

Lam D: Psychosocial family intervention in schizophrenia: a review of empirical studies. Psychol Med 21:423–441, 1991

Leff J, Kuipers L, Berkowitz R, et al: A controlled trial of social intervention in the families of schizophrenic patients. Br J Psychiatry 141:121–134, 1982

Lefley HP: Impact of mental illness in families of mental health professionals. J Nerv Ment Dis 175:613–619, 1987

Lukoff D, Nuechterlein KH, Ventura J: Symptom monitoring in the rehabilitation of schizophrenic patients. [See Appendix A: Manual for expanded Brief Psychiatric Rating Scale (BPRS).] Schizophr Bull 12:578–602, 1986

Marks I: Behavior therapy as an aid to self-care. Current Directions in Psychological Science 3:19–22, 1994

McFarlane WR, Dushay RA, Stastny P, et al: A comparison of two levels of family-aided assertive community treatment. Psychiatr Serv 47:744–750, 1996

Meltzer HY: Dimensions of outcome with clozapine. Br J Psychiatry 160 (suppl 17):46–53, 1992

Platt S: Measuring the burden of psychiatric illness on the family: an evaluation of some rating scales. Psychol Med 15:383–393, 1985

Platt S, Weyman A, Hirsch S, et al: The Social Behaviour Assessment Schedule (SBAS): rationale, contents, scoring and reliability of a new interview schedule. Social Psychiatry 15:43–55, 1980

Salleh MR: The burden of care of schizophrenia in Malay families. Acta Psychiatr Scand 89:180–185, 1994

Schene AH, Tessler RC, Gamache GM: Instruments measuring family or caregiver burden in severe mental illness. Soc Psychiatry Psychiatr Epidemiol 29:228–240, 1994

Slade PD, Bentall R: Psychological treatments for negative symptoms. Br J Psychiatry 155:133–135, 1989

Spaniol L, Jung H, Zipple AM: Families as a central resource in the rehabilitation of the severely psychiatrically disabled: report of a national survey (unpublished manuscript). Boston, MA, Boston University Center for Rehabilitation Research and Training in Mental Health, 1984

Sparrow SS, Balla DA, Cicchetti DV: Vineland Adaptive Behavior Scales. Circle Pines, MN, American Guidance Service, 1984

Stevens BC: The role of fluphenazine decanoate in lessening the burden of chronic schizophrenics in the community. Psychol Med 3:141–158, 1973

Veltro F, Magliano L, Lobrace S, et al: Burden on key relatives of patients with schizophrenia. Soc Psychiatry Psychiatr Epidemiol 29:66–70, 1994

Walker EF, Grimes KE, Davis D, et al: Childhood precursors of schizophrenia: facial expressions of emotion. Am J Psychiatry 150:1654–1660, 1993

Warner R: Recovery From Schizophrenia: Psychiatry and Political Economy. London, UK, Routledge & Kegan Paul, 1985

Willwerth J: Tinkering with madness. Time, August 1993, pp 40–42

Wing JK, Cooper JE, Sartorius N: The Description and Classification of Psychiatric Symptoms: An Instruction Manual for the PSE and CATEGO System. New York, Cambridge University Press, 1974

8 Regulatory Aspects of Drug Treatment for Negative Symptoms

Paul Bailey, M.R.C.Psych.

"...sooner or later, current sponsors of the positive/negative distinction will have to make up their minds in regards to the *nature of the link* between the symptoms named by these words." (Berrios 1991)

The task of a drug regulatory authority is defined clearly and succinctly in the United States Code of Federal Regulations (CFR): "[the U.S. Food and Drug Administration (FDA)] will approve an application after it determines that the drug meets the statutory standards for safety and effectiveness, manufacturing and controls, and labeling" (21 CFR Sec 314.105). The regulatory approach to negative symptoms thus requires consideration of how a drug treatment might be labeled and how efficacy and safety might be demonstrated. But as Berrios (1991) points out, such a discussion cannot be divorced entirely from a discussion of other aspects of schizophrenic symptomatology.

The original descriptions of schizophrenia by Bleuler (1911/1950) and Kraepelin (1919/1971) gave considerable weight to what would now be regarded as negative symptomatology—such as "autism" (withdrawal) and "affect" (including emotional blunting)—as well as to a progressive course of the illness, leading usually to severe handicap. Over time, these aspects came to be relatively neglected, and, especially in English-speaking circles, great importance became attached to the so-called first-rank symptoms of Schneider (1976). In the last decade or so, negative symptoms have been to some extent rediscovered, a number of rating scales have been devised to assess them, and the notion of first-rank symptoms has come under fire (e.g., Crichton 1996). Diagnostic criteria (American Psychiatric Association 1994) have been amended to give greater prominence to negative symptomatology. The concept of schizophrenia is not fixed, but changing: as Berrios (1991) noted, this is linked to our ignorance of the underlying pathophysiology of schizophrenia.

The efficacy of antipsychotic drugs in the treatment of positive symptoms of schizophrenia is beyond doubt. The efficacy of the same drugs in the treatment of negative symptoms has been the subject of controversy at least since Johnstone et al. (1978) failed to find an effect of flupenthixol on two core negative symptoms. The question as to whether negative symptoms respond to neuroleptic treatment remains open (for a review, see Carpenter 1996); I will argue that the answer depends on how the question is defined. Everyday clinical experience, however, strongly suggests that an unmet need exists for a better treatment for negative symptomatology.

In 1991, six clinical researchers from the European pharmaceutical industry who were engaged in the development of potential new treatments for negative symptoms met together to exchange ideas. We noted that no regulatory guidelines existed. After a review of the literature, we discussed our observations and concerns with hospital-based researchers in Europe, and an account of our deliberations was published (Möller et al. 1994). In this chapter, I shall develop some of the themes discussed in that paper with reference to subsequent regulatory authority decisions.

Negative Symptoms: Considerations for Clinical Trials

Among the points developed in the 1994 paper are the following:

1. There are several different definitions of the negative syndrome in schizophrenia (for a more detailed review, see Fenton and McGlashan 1992).
2. Secondary negative symptoms occurring during acute psychotic exacerbations need to be distinguished from "true" or "primary" negative symptoms, and also from depressive symptoms and drug-induced parkinsonism or sedation.
3. Therapeutic trials in the "negative symptom" indication show great methodological heterogeneity.

We therefore argued that such trials should exclude patients with high levels of positive symptoms, depressive symptoms, extrapyramidal side effects (EPS), and sedation and should require patients to show chronic "core" negative symptoms common to most classifications (namely, flat affect and poverty of speech). These proposals were purely pragmatic, intended to improve the methodology of clinical trials. We stated clearly that trial inclusion and exclusion criteria must not be too restrictive, or patient recruitment would become too difficult; for this reason, we avoided giving precise cutoff levels on various rating scales, which would in any case have been arbitrary. We were not proposing a new schizophrenic syndrome or attempting to [re]define "negative schizophrenia." The use of the word *considerations* in the title of the paper was intended to reflect this approach.

From a regulatory point of view, therefore, it could be argued that our work did not go far enough: we did not define a new diagnostic entity that could be used in labeling. And regulatory authorities (notably the FDA) have emphasized that they do not consider themselves responsible for the definition of clinical diagnostic entities. Nonetheless, clinical development of new neuroleptics has obliged regulatory agencies to address questions such as the following: What claims relating to negative symptoms can be made for new neuroleptics? What data are required to support such claims?

In the United States, the Psychopharmacologic Drugs Advisory Committee of the FDA has considered these issues in their discussions of new drug applications (NDAs) for risperidone and sertindole. The discussion on sertindole was devoted mainly to safety rather than efficacy issues; the comments made on negative symptoms were similar to those made for risperidone. Thus, risperidone will be used to illustrate the United States regulatory viewpoint.

The complicated evolution of a centralized NDA procedure in the European Community has been summarized by Kidd (1997). Briefly, in the centralized (or "concertation") procedure, the application is made directly to the European Agency for the Evaluation of Medicinal Products (European Medicines Evaluation Agency [EMEA]); the European Committee for Proprietary Medicinal Products (CPMP) then produces a European Public Assessment Report (EPAR) that is used as the basis for acceptance or refusal of the drug in all member states. To date, only one neuroleptic, olanzapine, has been submitted via the centralized procedure; the EPAR for olanzapine will be used to illustrate the European Community regulatory viewpoint.

The United States Position: Risperidone

In April 1993, the Psychopharmacologic Drugs Advisory Committee of the FDA met to discuss the NDA for risperidone. The proceedings of this meeting (U.S. Food and Drug Administration 1993) show that many of the issues addressed by the European working group were also discussed by this group of American experts at the invitation of FDA officials, who stated at the beginning of the meeting that the FDA does not "have a firm position or policy about negative symptoms" (U.S. Food and Drug Administration 1993, p. 65). Nonetheless, the FDA's concerns were clearly communicated (U.S. Food and Drug Administration 1993, p. 22):

- Is there agreement on what constitutes negative symptoms?
- Are negative symptoms part of the typical schizophrenic syndrome, or is it possible to tease out subtypes of schizophrenia that are predominantly characterized by negative symptoms? If so, should those subtypes be studied specifically?
- How should a regulatory agency handle claims for negative symptoms? ("Is this a legitimate claim or is this pseudo-specific in some sense?" [U.S. Food and Drug Administration 1993, p. 22])
- Is there evidence for differential responsiveness across neuroleptics with regard to negative symptoms?

The conclusions of the Psychopharmacologic Drugs Advisory Committee were very similar to those of the European working group. To establish a "negative symptom indication," one should study "a particular population" (U.S. Food and Drug Administration 1993, p. 282)–i.e., "a group of patients who have prominent negative symptoms" (p. 292), "a population of schizophrenics where positive symptoms are held constant in some way" (p. 293). An acutely ill population is not suitable "because in these populations very often the negative symptoms may be masked or complicated, or confounded by other things such as EPS" (p. 294).

Regarding optimal study duration, the European group, recognizing the lack of available data, tentatively suggested 8 weeks as "prudent." The United States group regarded 6 weeks to 8 weeks as insufficient (U.S. Food and Drug Administration 1993, pp. 295, 317), albeit without citing data, and one member hesitantly recommended 3 months (p. 295). Another suggested that in addition to the change in negative symptoms per se, the effects of that change on "jobs, social networks, reintegration into family" might be studied, over a period of "3 months, or 6 months, or 8 months" (p. 304).

Because the risperidone registration dossier did not contain a study aimed specifically at establishing the drug's efficacy for negative symptoms, the "negative symptom indication" was not accepted. However, it is interesting to note that a subsequent reanalysis of the risperidone data set by Schooler (1994) suggested that if the analysis were restricted to patients with predominantly negative symptomatology, an advantage for risperidone over haloperidol would be seen. This advantage was seen in change from baseline in the Positive and Negative Syndrome Scale (PANSS; Kay et al. 1987) total score, as well as in change in the Negative Syndrome Scale score, but became much less apparent when the whole data set (including patients with prominent positive symptoms) was considered. This analysis may be viewed as supporting the position of the European working group.

Nonetheless, it may be thought unfortunate that the FDA position on negative symptoms has still not been clearly stated, but rather must be deduced from the deliberations of the Advisory Committee. Although the FDA has clearly rejected the claim that risperidone has superior efficacy for negative symptoms, its view as to how this claim might be established remains undefined. A crucial element of study design—duration—remains entirely open; no evidence defining the minimum duration of a "negative symptom" study has ever been presented, and it is still unclear whether the measurement of effects of negative symptoms on social functioning is a central element of such a study or merely an optional extra.

The European Position: Olanzapine

The position of the CPMP concerning negative symptoms has to some extent been clarified by the marketing authorization for olanzapine (Committee for Proprietary Medicinal Products 1996). The indication finally approved was "treatment of schizophrenia," although a further paragraph contains information on olanzapine's effect on "associated depressive symptoms." Concerning negative symptoms, the authorization stated:

> The main studies showing statistically significant improved efficacy for these [i.e., negative] symptoms . . . were not done prospectively with relief of negative symptoms as the primary endpoint in a specific population of patients showing persistent negative symptomatology. (Committee for Proprietary Medicinal Products 1996, p. 16)

Concerning a study apparently showing that olanzapine had a greater effect than haloperidol on negative symptoms, the document argued:

> as the haloperidol doses were possibly too high (mean modal maintenance dose 11.8 mg) and could potentially induce depression mimicking negative

symptoms, it is difficult to conclude that olanzapine is undoubtedly more efficacious on negative scores than haloperidol. (Committee for Proprietary Medicinal Products 1996, p. 15).

This decision was based on the input of an "ad hoc expert working group," which reported that

> In order to claim a specific indication for negative symptoms, prospectively designed studies should be carried out in patients with stable schizophrenia who have prominent and persistent negative symptoms. As far as the negative symptoms in acute schizophrenia are concerned it would not be appropriate to mention a treatment effect in the Indications section of the Summary of Product Characteristics (SPC). (CPMP Efficacy Working Party and Ad Hoc Group of Experts on Schizophrenia joint meeting: minutes. London, June 7, 1996)

This ad hoc group came to a very similar conclusion concerning the indication "depressive symptoms in schizophrenia": "data should be gathered from studies prospectively designed to assess the effects in schizophrenic patients with clinically prominent depressive symptoms" (CPMP Efficacy Working Party and Ad Hoc Group of Experts on Schizophrenia, June 7, 1996). However, although "depressive symptoms in schizophrenia" was not accepted as an indication for olanzapine, relevant data are given in Section 4.1.2, "Further information on clinical data," in the SPC (Committee for Proprietary Medicinal Products 1996, p. 22), whereas no such data are given for negative symptoms. This discrepancy is difficult to explain, especially in view of the fact that a potential depressogenic action of other neuroleptics (haloperidol) is specifically mentioned in the marketing authorization.

Also of interest in this connection is the abbreviated prescribing information appearing in publicity for olanzapine in the United Kingdom. After mentioning the drug's effect on depressive symptoms, the prescribing information continues: "olanzapine was associated with significantly greater improvements in both negative and positive schizophrenic symptoms than placebo or comparator in most studies." Thus, the British authorities appear to have accepted the "negative symptom indication" that was explicitly rejected by the CPMP. It is noteworthy that this indication does not appear in the abbreviated prescribing information for clozapine, despite the existence of similar data comparing clozapine with chlorpromazine. Perhaps it was felt that the clozapine indication "treatment-resistant schizophrenia" already implied superior efficacy.

Thus, the theoretical standpoint of the CPMP is coherent, but its decisions are not. For both depressive and negative symptoms in schizophrenia, the CPMP wants to see prospective studies in appropriately defined populations. This is laudable as far as it goes—which, however, is not far enough: the CPMP's definition of the population for negative symptoms is even looser than that proposed by the European working group. In the absence of such studies, the CPMP has allowed labeling information relating to depressive but not negative symptoms, which is hard to understand. It is difficult to escape the conclusion that the European authorities, like the American ones, are worried about the potential commercial advantage given to the first compound to receive the "negative symptom" indication.

Furthermore, the British authorities appear to have accepted an indication not accepted by the CPMP, which would seem to weaken the concept of a pan-European drug approval process. This has unpalatable implications not only for this centralized European procedure but also, by implication, for the ongoing struggle for regulatory "globalization," the inherent problems of which are trenchantly addressed by Kidd (1997).

Discussion

A pharmaceutical company considering the development of a new compound in the indication "negative symptoms of schizophrenia" faces several daunting obstacles.

One such obstacle is the almost total lack of clear regulatory guidance concerning this indication. True, a consensus has emerged that clinical trials aimed at establishing a treatment effect on negative symptoms need to study a selected population, and regulatory authorities in Europe and the United States have accepted the methodological arguments against studying an acutely ill group of psychotic patients with prominent positive symptoms. However, these authorities have offered virtually no coherent advice about the kinds of studies they would like to see in support of the indication. What they do *not* want is clear; what they *do* want remains frustratingly obscure. This unsatisfactory state of affairs can only hinder the development of new treatments for these difficult and disabling symptoms.

However, even with the very limited guidance available, some practical obstacles become apparent. The "patients with stable schizophrenia who have prominent and persistent negative symptoms" demanded by the CPMP ad hoc working group are probably hard to find, even if fairly wide criteria are applied. In a study of the effect of amisulpiride and haloperidol on negative symptoms (Speller et al. 1997), patients on 18 medium- to long-stay wards in two psychiatric hospitals were screened; of 223 patients meeting DSM-III-R (American Psychiatric Association 1987) criteria for schizophrenia, only 60 (27%) were selected to enter the study on the basis of the criteria suggested by Möller et al (1994). As a result of the small sample size, the differences between the two treatments did not reach statistical significance. In addition, as the authors pointed out, "the findings should only be generalized with caution to the majority of patients with schizophrenia" (Speller et al. 1997, p. 567). To obtain a sample of sufficient size to deliver the necessary statistical power to demonstrate superiority over a conventional neuroleptic, a trial of a new treatment for negative symptoms will probably need to screen a very large patient population.

Another obstacle, as noted at the very start of this chapter, is the lack of a clear definition of the term "negative symptoms" and of the relationship of negative symptoms with the rest of the schizophrenia syndrome. The FDA has expressed its doubts thus:

> If you find it is unnecessary and redundant to say that an anti-psychotic has an effect on negative symptoms, [then] allowing one group to describe negative symptoms in some unique way creates the image of something being distinct and unique…when in fact it is not.…In the absence of evidence that is *compelling or convincing or substantial [my emphasis]*…that there is a differential effect of two drugs, what do you gain by saying anything about negative symptoms? (U.S. Food and Drug Administration 1993, pp. 309, 318)

The demand for "compelling" evidence reflects another regulatory concern (U.S. Food and Drug Administration 1993, p. 302): that the first drug approved with a specific negative symptom indication will have a substantial commercial advantage. Thus, by implication, the standards of proof required will be high. In view of the potential rewards, the interest shown by the pharmaceutical industry in the negative symptom indication is understandable. However, the potential difficulties of achieving the required standards of proof should not be underestimated.

References

American Psychiatric Association: Diagnostic and Statistical Manual of Mental Disorders, 3rd Edition, Revised. Washington, DC, American Psychiatric Association, 1994

American Psychiatric Association: Diagnostic and Statistical Manual of Mental Disorders, 4th Edition. Washington, DC, American Psychiatric Association, 1994

Berrios GE: Positive and negative signals [sic]: a conceptual history, in Negative Versus Positive Schizophrenia. Edited by Marneros A, Andreasen NC, Tsuang MT. Berlin, Germany, Springer-Verlag, 1991, p 17

Bleuler E: Dementia Praecox or the Group of Schizophrenias (1911). Translated by Zinkin J. New York, International Universities Press, 1950

Carpenter WT Jr: The treatment of negative symptoms: pharmacological and methodological issues. Br J Psychiatry 168 (suppl 29):17–22, 1996

Committee for Proprietary Medicinal Products: European Public Assessment Report: Zyprexa (olanzapine). Document CPMP/646/96. London, UK, European Medicines Evaluation Agency, 1996 (http://www.eudra.org/emea/pdfs/CPMP_EPAR_646_96.pdf)

Crichton P: First-rank symptoms or rank-and-file symptoms? Br J Psychiatry 169:537–540, 1996

Fenton WS, McGlashan TH: Testing systems for assessment of negative symptoms in schizophrenia. Arch Gen Psychiatry 49:179–184, 1992

Johnstone EC, Crow TJ, Frith CD, et al: Mechanism of the antipsychotic effect in the treatment of acute schizophrenia. Lancet 1:848–851, 1978

Kay SR, Fiszbein A, Opler LA: The Positive and Negative Syndrome Scale (PANSS) for schizophrenia. Schizophr Bull 13:261–276, 1987

Kidd D: The International Conference on Harmonization of Pharmaceutical Regulations, the European Medicines Evaluation Agency, and the FDA. Indiana Journal of Global Legal Studies 14(1):183–206, 1997 (http://www.law.indiana.edu/glsj/vol4/no1/kidpgp.html)

Kraepelin E: Dementia Praecox and Paraphrenia (1919). Translated by Barclay RM. Huntingdon, NY, RE Krieger, 1971

Möller HJ, Van Praag HM, Aufdembrinke B, et al: Negative symptoms in schizophrenia: considerations for clinical trials. Working group on negative symptoms in schizophrenia. Psychopharmacology (Berl) 115:221–228, 1994

Schneider K: Klinische Psychopathologie, 11th Edition. Stuttgart, Thieme, 1976, p 135

Schooler NR: Negative symptoms in schizophrenia: assessment of the effect of risperidone. J Clin Psychiatry 55 (5, suppl):22–28, 1994

Speller JC, Barnes TRE, Curson DA, et al: One-year, low-dose neuroleptic study of in-patients with chronic schizophrenia characterised by persistent negative symptoms. Br J Psychiatry 171:564–568, 1997

U.S. Food and Drug Administration: Psychopharmacologic Drugs Advisory Committee, Center for Drug Evaluation and Research, meeting 37 (April 29, 1993). Rockville, MD, U.S. Food and Drug Administration, 1993

The Biology and Pathophysiology of Negative Symptoms

Del D. Miller, Pharm.D., M.D.
Rajiv Tandon, M.D.

During the past 20 years, there has been a resurgence of interest in the negative symptoms associated with schizophrenia. Negative symptoms are currently considered to be a fundamental feature of the disease process and thought to be at least in part responsible for the social and occupational dysfunction seen in persons with schizophrenia. These realizations have produced a massive effort to identify the pathophysiology of negative symptoms, with an expectation that such a finding would lead to more effective treatments and ultimately provide relief for individuals suffering from schizophrenia. While this increasing research effort has allowed us to make great strides in our understanding of the neurobiological basis of negative symptoms, finding a single pathophysiology to account for all negative symptoms has remained elusive.

Much of the impetus for empirical research on negative symptoms of schizophrenia over the past two decades can be attributed to the work of Crow (1980), and Andreasen and Olsen (1982). In an effort to better understand schizophrenia and the neurobiology involved in the various symptoms, Crow (1980) suggested that schizophrenia could be categorized into two types. Originally, Crow suggested that type II (negative) schizophrenia was a later stage of schizophrenic illness, into which some patients with type I (positive) schizophrenia might progress; he subsequently (Crow 1985) revised this concept to propose that positive and negative symptoms reflected two relatively independent pathophysiological processes that could coexist in patients. He now postulated that the *type I* schizophrenic process was related to dopaminergic hyperactivity and responded well to treatment with antipsychotic medications that block postsynaptic D_2 dopamine (DA) receptors; in contrast, the *type II* schizophrenic process was considered to be related to structural brain abnormalities (e.g., enlarged ventricles) and possible dopaminergic hypofunction, reflecting a more degenerative condition or a developmental impairment. Andreasen and Olsen (1982) originally suggested that positive and negative symptoms in schizophrenia were dichotomous and defined two distinct types of schizophrenia patients (i.e., positive symptom patients and negative symptom patients) who likely had unique pathophysiologies. A subsequent study (Andreasen et al. 1990b) found that the vast majority of patients have both positive and negative symptoms and that categorizing patients as either positive or negative symptom patients appears to be of limited utility in differentiating possible differences in neurobiological mechanisms.

A major obstacle to a more complete understanding of the pathophysiology of negative symptoms is the fact that many different factors in schizophrenia can contribute to their phenotypic expression—that is, cross-sectionally primary and secondary negative symptoms can be indistinguishable in terms of their expression (Carpenter 1991; Sommers 1985; Tandon and Greden 1990). Carpenter et al. (1988) emphasized the need to differentiate between primary and secondary negative symptoms in order to understand the pathophysiology of primary negative symptoms. They suggested that although the exact pathophysiology of primary negative symptoms was unknown, it was likely related to neurotransmitter deficiency and/or frontal lobe dysfunction. Although the distinction between primary and secondary negative symptoms is important and makes intuitive sense, whether one can reliably differentiate between primary and secondary negative symptoms is debatable (Flaum and Andreasen 1995).

Implicit in Carpenter's distinctions between primary and secondary negative symptoms was the notion that secondary negative symptoms are brought about by positive symptoms, depression, extrapyramidal side effects (EPS) of antipsychotic medications, and lack of stimulation in the environment and thus involve different pathophysiological processes. Various investigators (Andreasen et al. 1994; Berman and Weinberger 1990; Bermanzohn and Siris 1992; Tandon and Greden 1989; Tandon et al. 1991a) have pointed out that even though positive symptoms, depression, and EPS can each separately produce phenotypically negative symptoms, it is possible that all of these etiological factors act via a common pathophysiological mechanism (Figure 9–1).

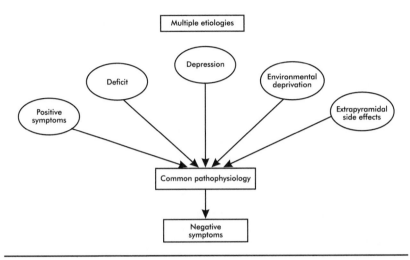

FIGURE 9–1. Model of multiple etiologies and a single pathophysiological mechanism underlying negative symptoms.

On the other hand, it is also possible that all negative symptoms arise from different pathophysiological pathways that converge in a final clinical consequence (Figure 9–2). In this model, mechanisms such as hypodopaminergic activity in frontal lobes, cholinergic excess, overactivity of the 5-hydroxytryptamine (5-HT [serotonin]) 2A receptor, and hypoglutamatergic activity may all lead to the production of negative symptoms. Conceivably, there may be a specific pathophysiological pathway that mediates negative symptoms for each single etiology; alternatively, different etiologies may all produce negative symptoms via multiple nonspecific pathophysiological processes.

Before embarking on a review of the specific neurobiological mechanisms implicated in the causation of negative symptoms, we present a brief summary of our current understanding of negative symptoms:

1. Negative symptoms constitute an integral component of schizophrenic psychopathology. They are not, however, specific to schizophrenia.
2. Data support the existence of a *negative symptom syndrome* that is distinct from a positive symptom syndrome in terms of clinical, prognostic, and neurobiological correlates (Robins and Guze 1970).
3. Positive and negative syndromes are *not mutually exclusive* and often coexist in the same patient.
4. Negative symptoms *are not a unitary construct*. They can be manifested as a consequence of a variety of conditions that occur over the course of

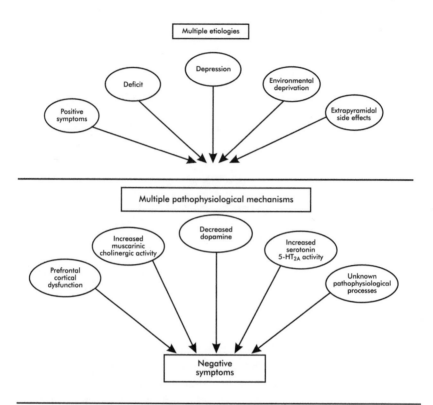

FIGURE 9–2.   Model of multiple etiological and multiple pathophysiological mechanisms underlying negative symptoms.

schizophrenic illness, such as core schizophrenic pathology, depression, or neuroleptic-induced EPS (Figure 9–3). Although distinguishing between these "etiological factors" may not be easy, awareness of different contributing factors provides a useful framework; results of studies investigating the neurobiological basis of negative symptomatology can be heavily influenced by the source of the negative symptoms. For instance, if one studies a group of schizophrenia patients with severe negative symptoms and the majority of these individuals concomitantly have significant depression, one may find neurobiological correlates of depression (i.e., reduced serotonergic activity) and mistakenly assume that these are components of negative symptom pathophysiology. The majority of the studies examining the neurobiology of negative symptoms have not made these distinctions, and this has led to discrepant findings.

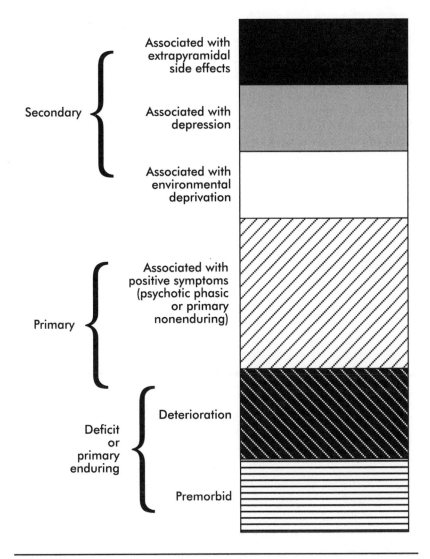

FIGURE 9–3. Components of negative symptoms.

5. From a *longitudinal perspective,* there appear to be three components of primary negative symptoms (Figure 9–4):

   a. a *premorbid component:* negative symptoms that are present before the first psychotic episode and that are associated with poor premorbid function

   b. a *psychotic-phasic or nonenduring component:* negative symptoms that oc-

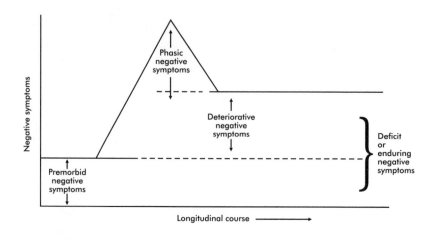

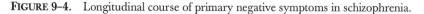

FIGURE 9–4.   Longitudinal course of primary negative symptoms in schizophrenia.

cur only in association with positive symptoms and that are restricted to the period around a psychotic exacerbation of schizophrenic
illness

c. a *postpsychotic deterioration component:* persistent negative symptoms that
occur after a psychotic episode and that reflect deterioration and decline from premorbid levels of functioning

It is not known whether the pathophysiological bases of these components of negative symptoms differ.

6. Negative symptoms *are not completely refractory to neuroleptic treatment.* In
fact, there is strong evidence that negative symptoms do improve over
the course of neuroleptic treatment; such improvement is most prominent in the acute phase of the illness. Clozapine and other atypical antipsychotics have generally been found to be more effective than
conventional neuroleptics in ameliorating negative symptoms (Jibson
and Tandon 1998; Meltzer et al. 1989); it appears that much of this
greater benefit may be related to their lower propensity to cause EPS.

Neurobiology of Negative Symptoms

Neuropharmacological, structural, and functional brain abnormalities have
all been implicated in the pathophysiology of negative symptoms in schizophrenia. The precise abnormal brain circuitry responsible for negative symp-

toms has not, however, been definitively defined; consequently, development of "negative symptom treatments" based on underlying putative mechanisms is still in a nascent stage.

Neuropharmacological Brain Abnormalities

Although viewing negative symptoms of schizophrenia as reflecting a neurotransmitter imbalance appears promising, clearly characterizing the specific neurotransmitter imbalances has been very difficult. Because antipsychotic medications—the first truly effective treatments for schizophrenia—appear to work by blocking dopamine neurotransmission, that neurotransmitter system has received the greatest interest. However, virtually every neurotransmitter, neuromodulator, or hormone discovered thus far has received consideration as being possibly implicated in the production of positive and negative symptoms of schizophrenia. Whereas positive symptoms can at least tentatively be explained as a consequence of either absolute or relative hyperdopaminergia, negative symptoms have been linked to several different kinds of neurotransmitter dysfunction.

Dopamine

Dopamine is the neurotransmitter most often implicated in the pathophysiology of schizophrenia. The dopamine hypothesis has been one of the bedrocks of schizophrenia pathophysiology ever since Carlsson and Lindquist (1963) reported that neuroleptics increased dopamine turnover in laboratory animals. Simply put, the hypothesis suggests that schizophrenia results, at least in part, from a functional overactivity or overabundance of dopamine in the brain. This speculation is supported by the fact that dopamine agonists such as L-dopa and amphetamine can cause psychosis (Angrist et al. 1973) and by the finding that all antipsychotic medications effective in treating positive symptoms block neurotransmission at the dopamine D_2 receptors. In contrast to their clear positive symptom efficacy, the effect of conventional antipsychotic medications on negative symptoms is more controversial. Although these agents have been shown to *decrease* negative symptoms during the acute psychotic phase of the illness, this result is likely related to their direct effect of reducing positive symptoms (e.g., hallucinations and delusions), which leads to an indirect reduction of negative symptoms (Tandon et al. 1990, 1993). Conversely, through their side effects (akinesia and akathisia), typical antipsychotics may *produce* affective flattening and avolition-apathy that mimic negative symptoms (Miller et al. 1994a). Therefore, the question of whether typical antipsychotics have a direct effect on the underlying pathophysiology of negative symptoms remains unresolved.

Although dopaminergic agonists can mimic positive symptoms such as paranoia and hallucinations reasonably well, they do not produce negative symptoms. Because it seems unlikely that simple hyperdopaminergia can account for both the positive and the negative symptoms of schizophrenia, several investigators have suggested that negative symptoms in schizophrenia may actually be related to *hypo*dopaminergic activity, particularly in the frontal regions (Berman and Weinberger 1990). Some investigators have found lower concentrations of cerebrospinal fluid (CSF) homovanillic acid (HVA) (presumably a measure of central dopaminergic activity) in association with greater severity of negative symptoms in persons with schizophrenia (Bowers 1974; Lindstrom 1985; Pickar et al. 1990). These findings could be compatible with a deficit of cortical dopamine activity in negative schizophrenia.

Weinberger and associates (1988), among others, have suggested that deficient mesocortical dopamine activity may contribute to the hypofrontality observed in many patients with schizophrenia, particularly those with severe negative symptoms (discussed in more detail below). In a Xenon-133 single-photon emission computed tomography (SPECT) study of drug-free schizophrenia patients selected for prominent "hypofrontality," Geraud and colleagues (1987) found that piribedil restored near-normal blood flow. Weinberger and co-workers (1988) found a positive correlation between CSF HVA concentrations and prefrontal regional cerebral blood flow (rCBF) in patients with schizophrenia during frontal cognitive activation with the Wisconsin Card Sorting Test (WCST; Heaton 1981). Daniel and colleagues have reported that both intravenous apomorphine (Daniel et al. 1989) and oral dextroamphetamine (Daniel et al. 1991) improved blood flow to the dorsolateral prefrontal cortex in patients performing the WCST.

If positive symptoms are in fact related to hyperdopaminergic activity and negative symptoms to hypodopaminergic activity, it seems counterintuitive to think that positive and negative symptoms could occur simultaneously in a given individual. Weinberger (1987) has proposed a neurodevelopmental model in which such an apparent dichotomy is possible. Various studies have demonstrated that there are complex feedback circuits between the prefrontal cortical and subcortical dopamine systems. Animal studies have found that a disruption of the dopamine system in the prefrontal cortex blocks feedback inhibition of the subcortical dopamine system, resulting in a functional hyperactivity of basal ganglia and limbic dopamine (Pycock et al. 1980). Weinberger (1987) suggested that in schizophrenia, increased subcortical dopamine activity is caused by diminished inhibitory effects of the hypoactive dopamine afferent projections from the prefrontal cortex. He proposed that a putative hypofunction of the prefrontal dopamine system provides a neurobiological basis for negative symptoms and that increased subcortical dopamine activity would account for positive symptoms. Thus, the combination of positive and negative symptoms in schizophrenia could potentially result from reduced prefrontal dopamine function (*negative symptoms*), leading to relative hyperactivity of subcortical dopamine (*positive symptoms*, consistent with the classical dopamine hypothesis).

As Pickar and co-workers (1990) pointed out, it is difficult to review pharmacological and metabolic studies of schizophrenia without concluding that dopamine plays a significant role in mediating both negative and positive symptoms. Nevertheless, the characteristics of dopaminergic involvement remain unclear. Likewise, the role that other dopamine receptors (e.g., D_1, D_3, D_4, D_5) play in schizophrenia—and particularly in the development and treatment of negative symptoms—remains ambiguous (Joyce and Meador-Woodruff 1997).

Serotonin

Early theories implicating serotonin in the pathogenesis of schizophrenia were based on the observation that lysergic acid diethylamide (LSD), a serotonin agonist, produced a psychosis with some features resembling schizophrenia. Interest in the role of the serotonin system in the negative symptoms of schizophrenia has been revived with the introduction of atypical antipsychotics (e.g., clozapine, risperidone, olanzapine, quetiapine, sertindole, ziprasidone), which are potent $5\text{-}HT_{2A}$ antagonists and have been shown to be effective in treating negative symptoms (Kane et al. 1988; Marder and Meibach 1994; Miller et al. 1994b; Small et al. 1997; Tandon et al. 1997; Tollefson and Sanger 1997; Tollefson et al. 1997; Zimbroff et al. 1997).

Some investigators have hypothesized that the atypical antipsychotics' superior efficiency in treating negative symptoms lies in their ability to block both dopaminergic (D_2) and serotonergic ($5\text{-}HT_2$) receptors centrally (Deutch et al. 1991; Meltzer 1989, 1991; Meltzer et al. 1989). Meltzer and others have suggested that the ratio of antagonism of $5\text{-}HT_2$ to dopamine D_2 receptors is the critical feature (Csernansky et al. 1990; Jibson and Tandon 1998; Meltzer 1989; Meltzer et al. 1989) that differentiates atypical from conventional antipsychotics. Although treatment studies with atypical antipsychotics may clarify the therapeutic effects of combined serotonin $5\text{-}HT_2$

and dopamine D_2 antagonism, they do not inform us about the absolute role of serotonin in the etiology of negative symptoms or about the potential benefit of pure 5-HT_2 antagonism in the treatment of negative symptoms. When combined with typical antipsychotics in patients with prominent negative symptoms in a double-blind, placebo-controlled trial, ritanserin (a potent 5-HT_2 antagonist) was found to induce a significant reduction in negative symptoms such as anergia and anxiety/depression (Gelders 1989). Selective serotonin reuptake inhibitors (SSRIs) have also been reported to improve positive and negative symptoms of schizophrenia when added to stable doses of conventional antipsychotics (Goff et al. 1990; Silver and Nassar 1992; Silver and Shmugliakov 1998). Although difficult to interpret, these findings may reflect the complexity of the serotonergic system (at least 14 different serotonin receptors have been identified) and the various interactions of the serotonin receptors with dopaminergic receptors. Another possibility is that these studies included heterogeneous samples of schizophrenic patients, some with primary and others with secondary negative symptoms, leading to conflicting results. Studies with large numbers of patients with negative symptoms secondary to depression may report finding improvement in negative symptoms during treatment with an SSRI antidepressant. Likewise, given that 5-HT_2 antagonism has been demonstrated to reduce EPS, potent 5-HT_2 blockers may produce improvement in secondary negative symptoms simply by reducing EPS).

Despite the pharmacological support for serotonin's role in the production of negative symptoms, few abnormalities of serotonin transmission in schizophrenia have been consistently replicated. However, studies that have examined 5-hydroxyindoleacetic acid (5-HIAA, a metabolite of serotonin) concentrations in the CSF have yielded interesting results. Four such studies found an inverse correlation between CSF 5-HIAA concentrations in schizophrenia and enlargement of cerebral ventricles (Jennings et al. 1984; Losonczy et al. 1986; Nyback et al. 1982; Potkin et al. 1983); increases in cerebral ventricular size have also been observed to be associated with prominent negative symptoms. Interestingly, lower 5-HIAA concentrations in patients with schizophrenia have also been found to be correlated with negative symptoms (Pickar et al. 1986) and with poor prefrontal activation during prefrontal neuropsychological tasks (Weinberger et al. 1988).

Thus, it appears that serotonin may play some role in the pathophysiology of negative symptoms of schizophrenia, although the precise nature of that role is currently unclear. Whether an abnormality in serotonin neurotransmission is the proximate cause of negative symptoms—or whether negative symptoms are related to serotonin's effect on dopamine activity in the ventral tegmental area (VTA) projection territories—remains unknown.

Acetylcholine

The cholinergic system has intermittently been implicated in the pathophysiology of schizophrenia, although the exact nature of its contribution remains poorly understood. Tandon and colleagues (1991a) have proposed that the cholinergic system plays a prominent role in the pathophysiology of schizophrenia and that cholinergic–dopaminergic interactions are relevant to the expression of positive and negative symptoms. Specifically, they have suggested that muscarinic hyperactivity may be relevant to the production of negative symptoms and that reduced cholinergic activity may be associated with positive symptoms (Tandon and Greden 1989). Tandon's group has shown that biperiden, a relatively specific M_1 antimuscarinic anticholinergic agent, significantly increases positive symptoms and reduces negative symptoms in medication-free patients with schizophrenia (Tandon et al. 1991a, 1992). In addition, there are numerous accounts of abuse of anticholinergic medications by schizophrenic patients; anticholinergic agents are reported to elevate mood, energize, stimulate, and improve socialization in persons with schizophrenia, regardless of whether they are taking antipsychotic medication (Fisch 1987; Tandon et al. 1988; Wells et al. 1989). Thus, it appears that these beneficial effects are not exclusively attributable to relief of EPS.

Another line of evidence suggesting a role for cholinergic activity in negative symptoms involves sleep regulation. Because the tonic and phasic aspects of dreaming or rapid eye movement (REM) sleep regulation are under cholinergic control, several groups have conducted sleep studies to elucidate the role of the cholinergic system in schizophrenia. Increased cholinergic activity is associated with REM latency and reduced slow-wave sleep. Studies have shown that the presence of negative symptoms is significantly correlated with shortened REM latency (Tandon et al. 1991a, 1992) and decreased slow-wave sleep (Ganguli et al. 1987; Tandon et al. 1989; van Kammen et al. 1988). Some recent studies (Riemann et al. 1994; Tandon 1999) have confirmed findings of increased cholinergic activity in the psychotic phase of schizophrenic illness.

Negative symptoms have also been linked with elevated postdexamethasone cortisol concentrations (Saffer et al. 1985; Tandon et al. 1991b) and increased growth hormone response to thyrotropin-releasing hormone (TRH) (Keshavan et al. 1989) and pyridostigmine (O'Keane et al. 1994) during the acute psychotic phase of schizophrenia. These data indirectly support the role of increased muscarinic activity in the production of negative symptoms in this phase of the illness, given that cholinergic mechanisms are known to play a significant role in releasing corticotropin-releasing hormone (CRH) and regulating the growth hormone response to TRH.

In addition, clozapine and olanzapine, two newer atypical antipsychotics with potent anticholinergic activity, have been reported to be more effective than traditional antipsychotics in reducing negative symptoms (Kane et al. 1988; Tollefson and Sanger 1997; Tollefson et al. 1997). Although other pharmacological mechanisms (e.g., serotonergic blockade, selective mesolimbic dopamine blockade) have been proposed as explanations for clozapine's and olanzapine's greater efficacy against negative symptoms, these agents' strong antimuscarinic activity must also be considered as a possible mechanism (Tandon 1999).

Thus, it appears that cholinergic hyperactivity may be involved in the production of negative symptoms in a subgroup of patients with schizophrenia; alternatively, cholinergic interactions with other neurotransmitter systems may be important in the pathogenesis of negative symptoms in certain phases of the illness.

Glutamate

An important role for glutamate in the pathogenesis of schizophrenia—and of negative symptoms in particular—is suggested by the strong resemblance between the psychiatric symptoms produced by administering phencyclidine (PCP) and features of schizophrenic illness (Domino and Luby 1981; Krystal et al. 1994; Lahti et al. 1995). PCP elicits both positive and negative symptoms, as well as cognitive impairment. Individuals exposed to PCP develop auditory and visual hallucinations, persecutory ideation, bizarre delusions, withdrawal, poverty of speech and thought, and catatonia. PCP is a glutamate *N*-methyl-D-aspartate (NMDA) receptor antagonist that produces a functional glutamate deficiency by blocking the NMDA glutamate receptor at the MK-801 site. Glutamate is the primary excitatory neurotransmitter for cortico-cortical, cortical–basal ganglial, and cortico-limbic connections (Carlsson 1995; Lund et al. 1975).

Decreased concentrations of glutamate in the CSF of patients with schizophrenia was reported by Kim and colleagues (1982), but this finding has not been replicated by other investigators (Gattaz et al. 1982; Perry 1982). Using synaptosomal preparations from postmortem brain tissue from persons with schizophrenia, Sherman and co-workers (1991a, 1991b) observed deficient glutamate release with veratridine-induced depolarization and on exposure to NMDA or kainic acid. Postmortem studies examining glutamate binding in brain tissue of persons with schizophrenia have had inconsistent findings (Kerwin et al. 1990).

Probably the strongest support for a role of glutamate hypofunction in negative symptoms has come from pharmacological trials, which have found that glutamate agonists (i.e., glycine and d-cycloserine) can improve negative symptoms when added to conventional antipsychotics. In the first double-blind, placebo-controlled trial of glycine added to conventional antipsychotics, Javitt and colleagues (1994) observed that glycine (0.4 g/kg/day) produced a significantly greater decrease in negative symptoms (as indicated by Positive and Negative Syndrome Scale [PANSS; Kay et al. 1987] scores) than was seen with placebo. This research group also reported a subsequent trial—a double-blind, placebo-controlled, randomly assigned, crossover design—in which glycine (0.8 g/kg/day) was added to patients' existing antipsychotic regimens (Heresco-Levy et al. 1996). They again found that adjuvant glycine induced significantly greater improvements in negative symptoms than did placebo. A recent study by Goff and colleagues (1995) also found that d-cycloserine, a partial agonist at the glycine site of the NMDA receptor, may improve negative symptoms in schizophrenia when added to conventional antipsychotic agents.

Because it is possible that glutamate abnormalities may be related to abnormal feedback (control) from other neurotransmitters, further research is needed to determine whether glutamate abnormalities in schizophrenia arise as a primary feature of schizophrenia or in response to abnormalities in other neurotransmitter systems.

Other Neurotransmitters

Other neurotransmitters and neuropeptides, such as norepinephrine (van Kammen et al. 1990) and cholecystokinin (Roberts et al. 1983), have also been implicated in the etiology of negative symptoms. Hypotheses proposing that abnormalities of a single neurotransmitter may be etiologically responsible for negative symptoms appear to be outdated. Whereas dopaminergic mechanisms may be important in the development of negative symptoms, serotonergic, cholinergic, glutamatergic, and noradrenergic mechanisms have also been linked with negative symptoms, and other neurotransmitters may be involved as well. Exactly how these systems interact remains unclear, and at this time, none of the proposed mechanisms can be considered definitive.

Although we often speak of the various neurotransmitter systems as if each exists in isolation, this is clearly not the case. Abnormalities or changes in a specific neurotransmitter system will have multiple effects on other neurotransmitter systems. For example, Kuroki and colleagues (1999) have shown that the atypical antipsychotics clozapine, risperidone, olanzapine, and amperozide, which are potent serotonin 5-HT_{2A} receptor antagonists, produce dopamine release in the prefrontal cortex. If hypodopaminergic activity is responsible for negative symptoms, a serotonin 5-HT_{2A} receptor antagonist may reverse the prefrontal hypodopaminergic state and effectively treat negative symptoms. Likewise, there are important interactions between and among the dopaminergic, serotonergic, cholinergic, glutamatergic, and noradrenergic transmitter systems. Another example of potential interactions between neurotransmitter systems, is the interaction between the dopaminergic and glutamatergic systems. Olney and Farber (1995) point out that one action of dopamine receptors is to inhibit glutamate release. Thus, a primary defect in the dopamine system that causes dopamine hyperactivity could result in excessive suppression of glutamate release at NMDA receptors, with consequent hypofunction of the NMDA receptor system as the basis for schizophrenic symptoms. One could speculate further that the combination of positive and negative symptoms in schizophrenia could result from hyperactivity of subcortical dopamine (positive symptoms) leading to hypofunction of the NMDA receptor system, which in turn could give rise to both positive and negative symptoms. Therefore, it is not surprising that an agent such as clozapine, which has been shown to block NMDA antagonist neurotoxicity, is effective in treating both positive and negative symptoms.

Structural and Functional Brain Abnormalities

In recent years there has been an enormous amount of research focusing on structural and functional brain imaging in schizophrenia. While the majority of studies have looked for abnormalities in schizophrenia in general, some have focused on abnormalities that are associated with particular symptom complexes such as negative symptoms.

Structural Brain Imaging

Although the findings of computed tomography (CT) and magnetic resonance imaging (MRI) studies have by no means been universally consistent, the majority of studies have shown a higher prevalence of structural brain abnormalities, particularly enlarged lateral ventricles, in schizophrenic patients with prominent negative symptoms (Andreasen 1982; Andreasen et al. 1990a, 1990c; Johnstone et al. 1976; Owens et al. 1985). In a review of 28 studies that examined whether negative symptoms are associated with structural brain abnormalities (enlarged ventricles), Marks and Luchins (1990) found that 18 of these studies provided some support for the model, while only 3 provided evidence in the opposite direction (i.e., positive symptoms were more strongly associated with brain abnormalities). Although few if any of these studies differentiated between primary and secondary negative symptoms, the consistency seen within these various patient samples suggest that negative symptoms are indeed associated with enlarged ventricles.

In an attempt to ascertain whether specific structural brain abnormalities are differentially related to positive, negative, and disorganized symptoms, Flaum and colleagues (1995) studied 166 subjects with schizophrenia and related disorders with volumetric measures of different brain regions of interest and correlated these volumetric measures with measures of psychopathology. They found that overall symptom severity was significantly correlated with larger lateral-ventricle volumes (lateral-ventricle, third-ventricle, and temporal horns) and smaller temporal lobe, hippocampal, and superior temporal gyral volumes. Negative symptom severity was significantly correlated with larger third-ventricle and smaller temporal lobe and hippocampal volumes. Because psychopathology ratings in this study were conducted when patients were off all psychoactive medications, it was unlikely that the negative symptoms were mimicked by antipsychotic-induced EPS. However, the negative symptoms could have been secondary to positive psychotic symptoms and/ or depression. An analysis of covariance relating each region of interest to the three symptom dimensions of negative, positive, and disorganized (and controlling for the other symptom dimensions) showed that both positive and negative symptom severity predicted increased third-ventricle volume. Thus, it seems likely that negative symptom severity is associated with enlarged third-ventricle volume.

Functional Brain Imaging

Recently, much research in schizophrenia has focused on functional neuroimaging. Functional neuroimaging depicts the *active* brain and assesses neurophysiological parameters such as cerebral circulation and neuronal metabolism. Current techniques include positron emission tomography (PET) and functional magnetic resonance imaging (fMRI). Using a variety of neuroimaging techniques, studies have found evidence suggesting that some people with schizophrenia may suffer from a specific dysfunction in the prefrontal cortex, sometimes described as "hypofrontality" (i.e., decreased metabolism or blood flow) (Andreasen et al. 1992, 1997; Buchsbaum et al. 1982; Weinberger et al. 1988).

Many studies that have used frontal activation tasks to examine clinical symptom severity have found that patients with the most severe negative symptoms show the greatest decrement in blood flow or metabolism in the prefrontal cortex with cognitive activation (Andreasen et al. 1992; Volkow et al. 1987; Wiesel et al. 1987). Volkow and co-workers (1987) observed that patients with negative symptoms ($n = 10$) had lower metabolism in the frontal lobes than patients with positive symptoms ($n = 8$) at rest, and that patients with positive symptoms showed greater frontal activation with a visual task than patients with negative symptoms. In a study of 15 medication-free patients with schizophrenia, Wiesel and associates (1987) reported that negative symptoms were negatively correlated with metabolism in the nucleus lenticularis, the prefrontal cortex, and the temporal cortex at rest. In one of the largest studies to examine hypofrontality in relation to negative symptoms, Andreasen and colleagues (1992) compared patients with chronic schizophrenia who had been off neuroleptics for 3 weeks ($n = 23$), patients with schizophrenia who had never received antipsychotic medications ($n = 15$), and healthy nonpsychiatrically ill volunteers ($n = 15$). rCBF was measured with Xenon-133 SPECT, and the Tower of London (Shallice 1982) was used as the frontal cognitive activating task. Andreasen et al. found that the normal volunteers showed a significant increase in left mesial frontal cortex blood flow with cognitive activation that was not seen in either the neuroleptic-naive or the chronic schizophrenia patients. Additionally, the decreased activation (relative to the healthy controls) was present only in the patients with high scores for negative symptoms.

This approach has been used by other groups to examine other symptom dimensions as well. Liddle and colleagues (1992) suggested that each of the three main schizophrenia syndromes (i.e., negative syndrome, reality distortion, and disorganization) are associated with a specific pattern of rCBF changes as measured by PET. These researchers found that psychomotor poverty (i.e., negative symptoms) was associated with decreased rCBF in the prefrontal and left parietal cortex and increased rCBF in the caudate nuclei; reality distortion was associated with decreased rCBF in the posterior cingulate and right caudate regions as well as increased rCBF in the left parahippocampal, the left ventral striatum, and the left prefrontotemporal regions; and disorganization was associated with decreased rCBF in the right temporoinsular-prefrontal cortices and increased rCBF in the right anterior cingulate.

Although the evidence is still not definitive, there is clearly a relationship between negative symptoms and "hypofrontality" in patients with schizophrenia. As mentioned above, many investigators have proposed that this hypofrontality may be related to hypodopaminergia in the frontal cortex; however, this remains a very tentative "working" theory requiring further research.

Conclusions

Negative symptoms remain a significant problem for many patients with schizophrenia. These symptoms are quite heterogeneous in nature, likely reflecting the multiple factors contributing to their presentation. It is possible that the various types of negative symptoms have very different underlying pathophysiologies—or, alternatively, that similar fundamental mechanisms create all types of negative symptoms. Although the distinction between primary and secondary negative symptoms is important for research on the neural mechanisms involved, it is probably of less clinical importance in terms of the daily impact on functioning for the affected individuals. That is, secondary negative symptoms are just as clinically disabling as primary negative symptoms. As far as individual patients are concerned, the fact that the newer medications may be more effective only for treating secondary negative symptoms—or that they cause fewer medication-induced symptoms—makes no difference; what matters to them is that they feel better and are less disabled.

The presenting negative symptoms could be a consequence of a variety of conditions that may arise in the longitudinal course of schizophrenia, such as worsening of core schizophrenic pathology, development of depression, or emergence of antipsychotic-induced EPS. Although distinguishing between these "etiological factors" may not be easy, awareness of different contributing factors is essential.

If these etiological factors act via a common pathophysiological mechanism, one would predict that an effective therapeutic modality would treat all negative symptoms. On the other hand, if the etiological factors arise from multiple pathophysiological pathways, one would expect that specific modalities would be effective in treating specific types of negative symptoms.

Many pathophysiological mechanisms for negative symptoms have been proposed, and there are data to support all of them. However, none of the these hypotheses can be considered definitive at present. Clearly, further research is needed to investigate the interactions between various neurotransmitters and to examine abnormalities in neural circuits in patients with prominent negative symptoms.

References

Andreasen NC: Negative symptoms in schizophrenia: definition and reliability. Arch Gen Psychiatry 39:784–788, 1982

Andreasen NC, Olsen SA: Negative vs. positive schizophrenia: definition and validation. Arch Gen Psychiatry 39:789–794, 1982

Andreasen NC, Ehrhardt JC, Swayze VW 2d, et al: Magnetic resonance imaging of the brain in schizophrenia: the pathophysiological significance of structural abnormalities. Arch Gen Psychiatry 47:35–44, 1990a

Andreasen NC, Flaum M, Swayze VW 2d, et al: Positive and negative symptoms in schizophrenia: a critical reappraisal. Arch Gen Psychiatry 47:615–621, 1990b

Andreasen NC, Swayze VW 2d, Flaum M: Ventricular enlargement in schizophrenia evaluated with computed tomographic scanning: effects of gender, age, and stage of illness. Arch Gen Psychiatry 47:1008–1015, 1990c

Andreasen NC, Rezai K, Alliger R, et al: Hypofrontality in neuroleptic-naive patients and in patients with chronic schizophrenia: assessment with Xenon 133 single-photon emission computed tomography and the Tower of London. Arch Gen Psychiatry 49:943–958, 1992

Andreasen NC, Nopoulos P, Schultz S, et al: Positive and negative symptoms of schizophrenia: past, present, and future. Acta Psychiatr Scand 90:51–59, 1994

Andreasen NC, O'Leary DS, Flaum M, et al: Hypofrontality in schizophrenia: distributed dysfunctional circuits in neuroleptic naive patients. Lancet 349(9067):1730–1734, 1997

Angrist BM, Sathananthan G, Gershon S: Behavioral effects of L-dopa in schizophrenic patients. Psychopharmacologia 31:1–12, 1973

Berman K, Weinberger D: Prefrontal dopamine and defect symptoms in schizophrenia, in Negative Schizophrenic Symptoms: Pathophysiology and Clinical Implications. Edited by Greden JF, Tandon R. Washington, DC, American Psychiatric Press, 1990, pp 83–95

Bermanzohn PC, Siris SC: Akinesia: a syndrome common to parkinsonism, retarded depression, and negative symptoms of schizophrenia. Compr Psychiatry 33:221–231, 1992

Bowers MB: Cortical dopamine turnover in schizophrenic syndromes. Arch Gen Psychiatry 31:50–54, 1974

Buchsbaum MS, Ingvar DH, Kessler R, et al.: Cerebral glucography with positron tomography. Arch Gen Psychiatry 39:251–259, 1982

Carlsson A: The dopamine theory revisited, in Schizophrenia. Edited by Hirsch SR, Weinberger DR. Oxford, UK, Blackwell Science, 1995, pp 379–400

Carlsson A, Lindquist M: Effect of chlorpromazine or haloperidol on formation of 3-methoxytyramine and normetanephrine in mouse brain. Acta Pharmacologica et Toxicologica 20:140–144, 1963

Carpenter WT Jr: Psychopathology and common sense: where we went wrong with negative symptoms. Biol Psychiatry 29:735–737, 1991

Carpenter WT Jr, Heinrichs DW, Alphs LD: Treatment of negative symptoms. Schizophr Bull 11:440–452, 1985

Carpenter WT Jr, Heinrichs DW, Wagman AMI: Deficit and nondeficit forms of schizophrenia: the concept. Am J Psychiatry 145:578–583, 1988

Crow TJ: Molecular pathology of schizophrenia: more than one disease process? BJM 280:66–68, 1980

Crow TJ: The two-syndrome concept: origins and current status. Schizophr Bull 11:471–486, 1985

Csernansky JG, King RJ, Faustman WO, et al: 5-HIAA in cerebrospinal fluid and deficit schizophrenic characteristics. Br J Psychiatry 156:501–507, 1990

Daniel DG, Berman KF, Weinberger DR: The effect of apomorphine on regional cerebral blood flow in schizophrenia. J Neuropsychiatry Clin Neurosci 1:377–384, 1989

Daniel DG, Weinberger DR, Jones DW, et al: The effect of amphetamine on regional cerebral blood flow during cognitive activation in schizophrenia. J Neurosci 11:1907–1917, 1991

Deutch AY, Moghaddam B, Innis RB, et al: Mechanisms of action of atypical antipsychotic drugs: implications for novel therapeutic strategies for schizophrenia. Schizophr Res 4:121–156, 1991

Domino EF, Luby E: Abnormal mental states induced by phencyclidine as a model of schizophrenia, in PCP (Phencyclidine): Historical and Current Perspectives. Edited by Domino EF. Ann Arbor, MI, NPP Books, 1981, pp 401–418

Fisch RZ: Trihexiphenidyl abuse: therapeutic implications for negative symptoms of schizophrenia. Acta Psychiatr Scand 75:91–94, 1987

Flaum M, Andreasen NC: The reliability of distinguishing primary versus secondary negative symptoms. Compr Psychiatry 36:421–427, 1995

Flaum M, O'Leary DS, Swayze VWI, et al: Symptom dimensions and brain morphology in schizophrenia and related psychotic disorders. J Psychiatr Res 29:261–275, 1995

Ganguli R, Reynolds CF, Kupfer DJ: Electoencephalographic sleep in young never-medicated schizophrenics. Arch Gen Psychiatry 44:36–44, 1987

Gattaz WF, Gatz D, Beckmann H: Glutamate in schizophrenics and healthy controls. Arch Psychiatr Nervenkr 231:221–225, 1982

Gelders YG: Thymosthenic agents, a novel approach in the treatment of schizophrenia. Br J Psychiatry 155:33–36, 1989

Geraud G, Arne-Bes MC, Guell A, et al: Reversibility of hemodynamic hypofrontality in schizophrenia. J Cereb Blood Flow Metab 7:9–12, 1987

Goff DC, Brotman AW, Waites M, et al: Trial of fluoxetine added to neuroleptics for treatment-resistant schizophrenic patients. Am J Psychiatry 147:492–494, 1990

Goff DC, Tsai G, Monoach DS, et al: Dose-finding trial of D-cycloserine added to neuroleptics for negative symptoms in schizophrenia. Am J Psychiatry 152:1212–1215, 1995

Heaton RK: The Wisconsin Card Sorting Test. Odessa, FL, Psychological Resources, 1981

Heresco-Levy U, Javitt DC, Ermilov M, et al: Double-blind, placebo-controlled, crossover trial of glycine adjuvant therapy for treatment-resistant schizophrenia. Br J Psychiatry 169:610–617, 1996

Javitt DC, Zylberman I, Zukin SR, et al: Amelioration of negative symptoms in schizophrenia by glycine. Am J Psychiatry 151:1234–1236, 1994

Jennings WS, Schultz, Narasimhacher N, et al: Brain ventricular size and CSF monoamine metabolite in an adolescent inpatient population. Psychiatry Res 16:87–94, 1984

Jibson MD, Tandon R: The new atypical antipsychotic medications. J Psychiatr Res 32:215–228, 1998

Johnstone EC, Crow TJ, Frith CD, et al: Cerebral ventricular size and cognitive impairment in chronic schizophrenia. Lancet 2:924–926, 1976

Joyce JN, Meador-Woodruff JH: Linking the family of D_2 receptors to neuronal circuits in human brain: insights into schizophrenia. Neuropsychopharmacology 16:375–384, 1997

Kane J, Honifeld G, Singer J, et al: Clozapine for the treatment-resistant schizophrenic: a double-blind comparison with chlorpromazine. Arch Gen Psychiatry 45:789–796, 1988

Kay SR, Fiszbein A, Opler LA: The Positive and Negative Syndrome Scale (PANSS) for schizophrenia. Schizophr Bull 13:261–276, 1987

Kerwin R, Patel S, Meldrum B: Quantitative autoradiographic analysis of glutamate binding sites in the hippocampal formation in normal and schizophrenic brain post mortem. Neuroscience 39:25–32, 1990

Keshaven MS, Brar J, Campbell K, et al: Growth hormone response to TRH and negative symptoms in schizophrenia. Biol Psychiatry 25:173–174, 1989

Kim JS, Kornhuber HH, Schmid-Burgk W, et al: Low cerebrospinal fluid glutamate in schizophrenic patients and a new hypothesis on schizophrenia. Neurosci Lett 20:379–382, 1982

Kuroki T, Meltzer HY, Ichikawa J: Effects of antipsychotic drugs on extracellular dopamine levels in rat medial prefrontal cortex and nucleus accumbens. J Pharmacol Exp Ther 288:774–781, 1999

Krystal JH, Karper LP, Seibyl JP, et al: Subanesthetic effects of the noncompetitive NMDA antagonist, ketamine, in humans: psychotomimetic, perceptual, cognitive, and neuroendocrine responses. Arch Gen Psychiatry 51:199–214, 1994

Lahti AC, Holcomb HH, Medoff DR, et al: Ketamine activates psychosis and alters limbic blood flow in schizophrenia. Neuroreport 6:869–872, 1995

Liddle PF, Friston KJ, Frith CD, et al: Patterns of cerebral blood flow in schizophrenia. Br J Psychiatry 160:179–186, 1992

Lindstrom LH: Low HVA and normal 5-HIAA CSF levels in drug free schizophrenic patients compared to healthy volunteers: correlations to symptomatology and family history. Psychiatry Res 14:265–273, 1985

Losonczy MF, Song IS, Mohs RC, et al: Correlates of lateral ventricular size in chronic schizophrenia: biological measures. Am J Psychiatry 143:1113–1118, 1986

Lund JS, Lund RD, Hendrickson AE, et al: The origin of efferent pathways from primary visual cortex, area 17, of the macaque monkeys as shown by retrograde transport of horseradish peroxidase. J Comp Neurol 164:287–303, 1975

Marder SR, Meibach RC: Risperidone in the treatment of schizophrenia. Am J Psychiatry 151:825–835, 1994

Marks RC, Luchins DJ: Relationship between brain imaging findings in schizophrenia and psychopathology: a review of the literature relating to positive and negative symptoms, in Schizophrenia: Positive and Negative Symptoms and Syndromes. Edited by Andreasen NC. Basel, Switzerland, Karger, 1990, pp 89–123

Meltzer HY: Clinical studies on the mechanism of action of clozapine: the dopamine-serotonin hypothesis of schizophrenia. Psychopharmacology (Berl) 99 (suppl): S18–S27, 1989

Meltzer HY: The mechanism of action of novel antipsychotic drugs. Schizophr Bull 17:263–286, 1991

Meltzer HY, Bastani B, Ramirez L, et al: Clozapine: new research on efficacy and mechanism of action. European Archives of Psychiatry and Neurological Sciences 238:332–339, 1989

Miller DD, Flaum M, Arndt S, et al: Effect of antipsychotic withdrawal on negative symptoms in schizophrenia. Neuropsychopharmacology 11:11–20, 1994a

Miller DD, Perry PJ, Cadoret RJ, et al: Clozapine's effect on negative symptoms in treatment-refractory schizophrenics. Compr Psychiatry 35:8–15, 1994b

Nyback H, Wiesel FA, Berggren BM: Computed tomography of the brain in patients with acute psychosis and in healthy volunteers. Acta Psychiatr Scand 65:403–414, 1982

O'Keane V, Abel K, Murray RM: Growth hormone responses to pyridostigmine in schizophrenia: evidence for cholinergic dysfunction. Biol Psychiatry 36:582–588, 1994

Olney JW, Farber NB: Glutamate receptor dysfunction and schizophrenia. Arch Gen Psychiatry 52:998–1007, 1995

Owens DGC, Johnstone EC, Crow TJ, et al: Lateral ventricular size in schizophrenia: relationship to the disease process and its clinical manifestations. Psychol Med 15:27–41, 1985

Perry TL: Normal cerebrospinal fluid and brain glutamate levels in schizophrenia do not support the hypothesis of glutamatergic neuronal dysfunction. Neurosci Lett 28:81–85, 1982

Pickar D, Roy A, Breier A, et al: Suicide and aggression in schizophrenia: neurobiological correlates. Ann N Y Acad Sci 189–196, 1986

Pickar D, Breier A, Hsiao J, et al: Cerebrospinal fluid and plasma monoamine metabolites and their relation to psychosis. Arch Gen Psychiatry 47:641–648, 1990

Potkin S, Weinberger DR, Linnoila M, et al: Low CSF 5-hydoxyindoleacetic acid in schizophrenic brains with enlarged ventricles. Am J Psychiatry 140:21–25, 1983

Pycock CJ, Kerwin RW, Carter CJ: Effect of lesion of cortical DA terminals on subcortical DA receptors in rats. Nature 286:74–77, 1980

Riemann D, Hohagen F, Krieger S, et al: Cholinergic REM induction test: muscarinic supersensitivity underlies polysomnographic findings in both depression and schizophrenia. J Psychiatr Res 28:195–210, 1994

Roberts GW, Ferrie IN, Lee Y, et al: Peptides, the limbic lobe and schizophrenia. Brain Res 288:199–211, 1983

Robins E, Guze SB: Establishment of diagnostic validity in psychiatric illness: its application to schizophrenia. Am J Psychiatry 126:983–987, 1970

Saffer D, Metcalfe M, Coppen A: Abnormal dexamethasone suppression test in type II schizophrenia? Br J Psychiatry 147:721–723, 1985

Shallice T: Specific impairments of planning. Philos Trans R Soc Lond B Biol Sci 298:199–209, 1982

Sherman AD, Davidson AT, Baruah S, et al: Evidence of glutamatergic deficiency in schizophrenia. Neurosci Lett 121:77–80, 1991a

Sherman AD, Hegwood TS, Baruah S, et al: Deficient NMDA-mediated glutamate release from synaptosomes of schizophrenics. Biol Psychiatry 30:1191–1198, 1991b

Silver H, Nassar A: Fluvoxamine improves negative symptoms in treated chronic schizophrenia: an add-on double-blind, placebo-controlled study. Biol Psychiatry 31:698–704, 1992

Silver H, Shmugliakov N: Augmentation with fluvoxamine but not maprotiline improves negative symptoms in treated schizophrenia: evidence for a specific serotonergic effect from a double-blind study. J Clin Psychopharmacol 18:208–211, 1998

Small JG, Hirsch SR, Arvanitis LA, et al: Quetiapine in patients with schizophrenia: a high- and low-dose double-blind comparison with placebo. Arch Gen Psychiatry 54:549–557, 1997

Sommers AA: "Negative symptoms": conceptual and methodological problems. Schizophr Bull 11:364–379, 1985

Tandon R: Cholinergic aspects of schizophrenia. Br J Psychiatry 173 (suppl 37):7–11, 1999

Tandon R, Greden JF: Cholinergic hyperactivity and negative schizophrenic symptoms. Arch Gen Psychiatry 46:745–753, 1989

Tandon R, Greden JF: Conclusion: is integration possible? in Negative Schizophrenic Symptoms: Pathophysiology and Clinical Implications. Edited by Greden JF, Tandon R. Washington, DC, American Psychiatric Press, 1990, pp 233–239

Tandon R, Greden JF, Silk KR: Treatment of negative schizophrenic symptoms with trihexyphenidyl. J Clin Psychopharmacol 8:212–215, 1988

Tandon R, Shipley J DeQuardo J, et al: Association between abnormal rapid eye movement sleep and negative symptoms in schizophrenia. Psychiatry Res 27:359–361, 1989

Tandon R, Goldman RS, Goodson J, et al: Mutability and relationship between positive and negative symptoms during neuroleptic treatment in schizophrenia. Biol Psychiatry 27:1323–1326, 1990

Tandon R, Greden JF, Goodson J, et al: Muscarinic hyperactivity in schizophrenia: relationship to positive and negative symptoms. Schizophr Res 4:23–30, 1991a

Tandon R, Mazzara C, DeQuardo JR, et al: Dexamethasone suppression test in schizophrenia: relationship to symptomatology, ventricular enlargement, and outcome. Biol Psychiatry 29:953–964, 1991b

Tandon R, DeQuardo JR, Goodson J, et al: Effects of anticholinergics on positive and negative symptoms in schizophrenia. Psychopharmacol Bull 28:297–302, 1992

Tandon R, Ribeiro SC, DeQuardo JR, et al: Covariance of positive and negative symptoms during neuroleptic treatment in schizophrenia: a replication. Biol Psychiatry 34:495–497, 1993

Tandon R, Harrington E, Zorn S: Ziprasidone: a novel antipsychotic with unique pharmacology and therapeutic potential. J Serotonin Research 4:159–177, 1997

Tollefson GD, Sanger TM: Negative symptoms: a path analytic approach to a double-blind, placebo- and haloperidol-controlled clinical trial with olanzapine. Am J Psychiatry 154:466–474, 1997

Tollefson GD, Beasley CM Jr, Tran PV, et al: Olanzapine versus haloperidol in the treatment of schizophrenia and schizoaffective and schizophreniform disorders: results of an international collaborative trial. Am J Psychiatry 154:457–465, 1997

van Kammen DP, van Kammen WB, Peters J, et al: Decreased slow-wave sleep and enlarged ventricles in schizophrenia. Neuropsychopharmacology 1:265–271, 1988

van Kammen DP, Peters J, Yao J, et al: Norepinephrine in acute exacerbations of chronic schizophrenia: negative symptoms revisited. Arch Gen Psychiatry 47:161–168, 1990

Volkow ND, Wolf AP, Van Gelder P, et al: Phenomenological correlates of metabolic activity in 18 patients with chronic schizophrenia. Am J Psychiatry 144:151–158, 1987

Weinberger DR: Implications of normal brain development for the pathogenesis of schizophrenia. Arch Gen Psychiatry 44:660–669, 1987

Weinberger D, Berman K, Zec RF: Physiological dysfunction of dorsolateral prefrontal cortex in schizophrenia, III: a new cohort and evidence for a monoaminergic mechanism. Arch Gen Psychiatry 45:609–615, 1988

Wells BG, Marken PA, Rickman LA, et al: Characterizing anticholinergic abuse in community mental health. J Clin Psychopharmacol 9:431–435, 1989

Wiesel FA, Wik G, Sjogren I, et al: Altered relationship between metabolic rates of glucose in brain regions of schizophrenic patients. Acta Psychiatr Scand 76:642–647, 1987

Zimbroff DL, Kane JM, Tamminga CA, et al: Controlled, dose-response study of sertindole and haloperidol in the treatment of schizophrenia. Am J Psychiatry 154:782–791, 1997

Index